GREEN LAND VEGETABLE COOKBOOK

Healthy, Delicious, Low-Carb Recipes for Weight Loss and Wellness

BONUS: 30 days meal plan for you

By

Yvette W. Messenger

Copyright

Disclaimer

The "Greenland Vegetable Cookbook" contains information that is intended solely for general educational purposes. Although every attempt has been made to guarantee the content's accuracy and completeness, the author disclaims all express and implied representations and warranties regarding the cookbook's content, information, recipes, and related graphics, as well as their availability, completeness, accuracy, suitability, and reliability. You are solely liable for any reliance you put on such information. The writer expressly disclaims all liability for any loss or damage, including but not limited to consequential or indirect loss or damage, bodily injury, or any cost, loss, or damage resulting from using the information in the "Greenland Vegetable Cookbook."

For specialised nutritional or health advice, it is recommended to speak with a licenced specialist. Any negative effects or repercussions arising from using the recipes or information in this cookbook are not the author's responsibility.
You accept these conditions by using this cookbook, and you understand that you are in charge of your own behaviour. The author disclaims any liability deriving from your use of the offered information and reserves the right to make modifications to the content.

About the Author

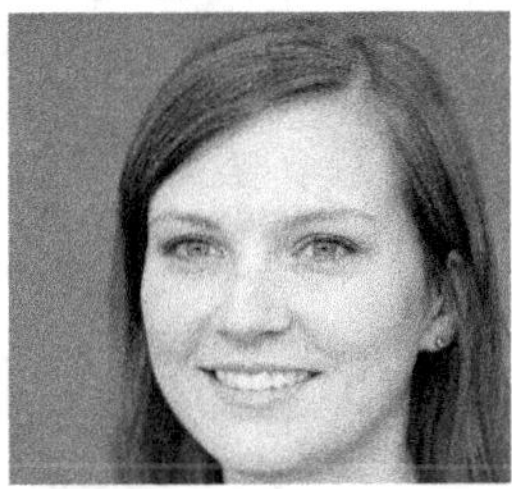

Meet Yvette W. Messenger, the culinary virtuoso and passionate advocate for healthy living. As an accomplished chef, Yvette brings her expertise to the forefront of the culinary world, weaving together her love for vegetarian diets, weight management, and the art of healthy eating.

Chef Yvette's Culinary Journey:

Yvette's culinary journey is a fusion of her love for nutritious, flavorful meals and her commitment to a lifestyle that promotes well-being. Her exploration of healthy living extends beyond the kitchen, reflecting a holistic approach to nourishing the body and soul.

Passion for Vegetarian Diets:

Yvette's heart lies in the vibrant world of vegetarian cuisine. Her recipes celebrate the diverse flavors and nutritional richness that vegetables bring to the table. Through her culinary creations, she aims to inspire others to embrace the goodness of plant-based eating, proving that health-conscious meals can be both delectable and satisfying.

Weight Watching Expertise:

As someone deeply invested in the well-being of others, Yvette understands the significance of weight management. Her culinary expertise extends to crafting dishes that align with weight-watching goals without compromising on taste. Yvette's recipes are a testament to the belief that healthy eating can be a joyful and flavorsome journey.

Healthy Eating Advocate:

Yvette is not just a chef; she's a dedicated advocate for healthy eating. Her commitment to this cause is evident in every page of the "Greenland Vegetable Cookbook," where she shares her knowledge, tips, and a treasure trove of recipes designed to make healthy eating an accessible and enjoyable lifestyle.

Join Yvette on the Path to Wellness:

Through her culinary creations, Chef Yvette W. Messenger invites you to join her on a journey to discover the joy of healthy living. Her approachable recipes, rooted in a passion for vegetarian diets, weight watching, and overall wellness, make the "Greenland Vegetable Cookbook" not just a collection of recipes but a guide to embracing a lifestyle that celebrates good food and good health.

Get ready to embark on a flavorful adventure guided by Yvette's expertise. May this cookbook inspire you to savor the richness of healthy eating and discover the artistry that comes with every delicious, nourishing dish. Welcome to the culinary world of Yvette W. Messenger!

BONUS: 30 days meal plan

Hello, wellness warrior! Congratulations on taking the first step towards a healthy lifestyle with the "Greenland Vegetable Cookbook." We're excited to put an extra bonus on top of your gastronomic trip!

Daily meal plans:

Welcome to our special "30 Days to a Healthier You" Meal Plan, which will take you on a 30-day journey of flavours, nutrition, and delectable discoveries. We've designed daily meal plans that are more than just food; they're a celebration of lively, health-conscious living. Let's have a look at what's in store for you each day:

Day 1 to 7: New Beginnings

Begin your journey with filling breakfasts such as avocado toast with poached eggs. Lunches feature colourful salads, and evenings feature robust vegetable stir-fries. Snack on crunchy vegetables and hummus for a midday pick-me-up.

Day 8-14: Protein-Rich Treats

Enjoy protein-packed breakfast bowls and grilled chicken salads as we go deeper. Baked salmon and vegetable medleys add a cosy touch to dinners. Nuts and seeds are an excellent source of energy therefore their perfect for a go-to snack

Day 15-21: Plant-Powered Happiness

Smoothie bowls for breakfast and quinoa-stuffed bell peppers for lunch are two ways to embrace plant-based bliss. Dinners become more daring with lentil curry, and for a wonderful twist, nibble on fruit slices or Greek yoghurt.

Day 22-28: Delicious Comfort

Breakfasts of muesli and fruit provide comfort. Soups are served for lunch, while turkey meatballs and roasted vegetables are served for dinner. For a sweet snack, grab a handful of berries or a tiny dish of dark chocolate.

Day 29-30: Culinary Showcase

Finish your journey on a high note with tasty yet healthy sweets. Consider sweet potato pancakes for breakfast, grilled prawn salads for lunch and a dinner worthy vegetable lasagna. Enjoy a modest portion of your favourite nutritious dessert

TABLE OF CONTENTS

INTRODUCTION

Welcome to the "Greenland Vegetable Cookbook," a culinary journey into the world of healthy, delicious, and low-carb recipes that not only tantalise your taste buds but also support your weight loss and overall wellness. This cookbook is designed with the novice cook in mind, making it easy for anyone to prepare mouthwatering meals using common vegetables found in your local grocery store.

In today's fast-paced world, maintaining a healthy lifestyle and managing your weight is more important than ever. This cookbook is your guide to embracing a diet rich in vegetables while reducing carbs, without compromising on flavour. We've carefully crafted each recipe to ensure that you can savour the goodness of Greenlandic vegetables and experience their natural tastes.

Our goal is to make your cooking journey as straightforward as possible. That's why we've provided standardised measurements for ingredients and kept the recipes simple, so beginners and experienced cooks alike can create these delectable dishes with ease.

Whether you're looking for appetisers to impress your guests, wholesome breakfasts to kickstart your day, satisfying lunches, or hearty dinners, we've got you covered. And when it's time for a sweet treat or a refreshing beverage, you'll find delightful options in our dessert and beverage chapters.

The recipes in this book are not only about culinary satisfaction but also about enhancing your well-being. We've incorporated low-carb principles to help you maintain or achieve your weight loss goals. Vegetables are your allies on this journey, offering an array of nutrients, textures, and flavours.

So, let's embark on this flavorful adventure together. Get ready to explore the bountiful world of Greenlandic vegetables and create dishes that will make your taste buds dance. Whether you're a beginner or a seasoned cook, you'll find inspiration and simplicity within these pages. Your path to a healthier, more delicious, and lower-carb lifestyle begins here. Enjoy the journey!

In this cookbook, we invite you to embrace the wonders of Greenlandic vegetables, which not only contribute to your well-being but also open the door to a world of culinary creativity. Vegetables are the foundation of our recipes, ensuring that each dish is not only healthy but also bursting with flavour and texture.

If you've ever thought that adopting a low-carb lifestyle meant sacrificing taste and satisfaction, this book is here to prove otherwise. We believe that a healthy diet should be a source of joy, not a source of deprivation. Our recipes are carefully designed to align with your weight loss goals while keeping your taste buds in mind.

The beauty of this cookbook lies in its versatility. Whether you're cooking for yourself, your family, or hosting a gathering, you'll find recipes suitable for any occasion. From the simplicity of vegetable stir-fries to the heartiness of roasted vegetables with herbed quinoa, we've curated a diverse selection of dishes to suit your needs.

At the heart of our approach is an appreciation for the natural flavours of vegetables. We encourage you to savour the freshness of produce readily available at your local grocery store. These common vegetables serve as the canvas for your culinary creations, allowing you to experiment, personalise, and make each recipe your own.

As you dive into the pages of this cookbook, you'll discover that a healthier, lower-carb lifestyle can be both achievable and delicious. Our aim is to provide you with the tools, knowledge, and inspiration to make informed choices about your diet while enjoying the incredible journey of preparing and savouring delectable meals. So, let's embark on this wholesome adventure together and redefine your approach to cooking and eating. Welcome to the "Greenland Vegetable Cookbook.

BASICS OF COOKING WITH COMMON VEGETABLES

1. Vegetable Selection:

- When you're choosing vegetables, consider what's in season. Seasonal veggies are not only fresher but often cheaper and more environmentally friendly.
- The key to selecting good vegetables is to look for firmness and vibrant colours. Avoid vegetables with soft spots, wilting, or discoloration.

2. Washing and Preparing:

- It's crucial to give your vegetables a thorough wash to remove dirt, bacteria, and any pesticide residues. Use a brush or your hands to clean them properly.
- As for preparing them, the goal is to ensure they're uniform in size for even cooking. Depending on your recipe, you may need to peel, chop, dice, or slice them.

3. Cutting and Slicing:

- Different recipes may require different cutting techniques. For instance, dicing is great for soups, while julienne works well for stir-fries. Slicing vegetables thinly is perfect for salads.
- Remember that the size of your cuts can affect cooking time, so choose accordingly.

4. Cooking Methods:

- The choice of cooking method can greatly influence the flavour and texture of your vegetables:
    - Steaming: Ideal for retaining the maximum nutrients and natural flavours.
    - Sautéing: A quick and versatile method that keeps the crunch in many veggies.
    - Roasting: This method enhances the sweetness and adds a delicious caramelised flavour.

- o Boiling: Perfect for making soups, stews, or blanching veggies.
- o Grilling: Gives vegetables a smoky flavour and those appealing grill marks.

5. Seasoning and Flavors:

- Playing with seasonings is one of the joys of cooking with vegetables. Experiment with herbs, spices, garlic, and different oils to bring out the best in each vegetable.
- Don't forget the importance of salt and pepper to balance the flavours, but use them sparingly to control your sodium intake.

6. Doneness:

- Achieving the right level of doneness is key to a successful vegetable dish. Overcooked vegetables can become mushy and unappetizing, while undercooked ones may be too tough to enjoy.
- To check doneness, try piercing your veggies with a fork or tasting them. They should be tender but not overly soft.

7. Combining Flavours:

- Part of the fun in working with common vegetables is the variety of combinations you can explore. Mixing textures, colours, and flavours can create captivating and balanced dishes.

8. Serving:

- Think about the best way to present your vegetables. They can be served hot, cold, or at room temperature, depending on the recipe and your preference.
- Garnishing with fresh herbs, grated cheese, a drizzle of olive oil, or a sprinkle of nuts can elevate the visual appeal and taste.

Now that you've learned more about the basics of cooking with common vegetables, you're equipped with the skills to create a wide array of delectable dishes. Experiment, have fun, and let your creativity shine in the kitchen as you make the most of these wholesome ingredients. Your culinary journey is just beginning, so enjoy the process and savour the incredible flavours that common vegetables bring to your table!

Chapter 1: Appetising Appetisers

1.EASY BAKE BRIE RECIPE

Prep time: 5 minutes

Cook time: 40 minutes

Total time: 55 minutes

Serving: 7-8

Ingredients

- 1 12-14 oz wheel of brie
- 1/2 tsp. chopped fresh thyme leaves
- 1/2 tsp. chopped fresh rosemary leaves
- 2 tbsp. honey
- Sea salt, optional
- Toasted bread, apple slices, and/or grapes, for serving

Directions

•Take the brie out of the fridge. Take off the paper covering and either put the wheel back in the bottom of the wooden box it came in or set it on a little piece of parchment paper, somewhat bigger than the brie wheel itself. Cut criss cross-shaped, extremely shallow slits every ½ to 1 inch over the top of the brie, just through the rind layer. Allow to stand at room temperature for half an hour.

•Set oven temperature to 350 degrees. The brie should be put on a little sheet tray. Drizzle with honey and scatter the fresh thyme and rosemary over top. Bake until very soft, 20 to 25 minutes.

• Gently move the brie to a serving platter, keeping it either in the box or on the parchment paper.

2.EGGPLANT CAPONATA

Prep time: 20 minutes

 Cook time: 40 minutes

Total time: 1hour

Serving: 5

Ingredients

- 1 large eggplant, cut into 1-inch cubes

- 1 red bell pepper, cut in quarters, core and seeds removed

- 1/4 c. olive oil, divided

- 2 tsp. kosher salt, divided

- 1 tsp. freshly ground black pepper, divided

- 1 medium yellow onion, diced

- 2 stalks celery, diced

- 4 garlic cloves, finely chopped

- 1 tsp. dried oregano

- 1 14-ounce can crushed tomatoes

- 1/2 c. pitted green olives, coarsely chopped

- 1/3 c. golden raisins

- 3 tbsp. red wine vinegar

- 2 tbsp. capers, drained

- 1 tbsp. granulated sugar

- 1/4 c. chopped fresh parsley

- Toasted bread, to serve

Directions

•Set oven temperature to 425°F. Line baking sheet with parchment paper

•Place the bell pepper and eggplant on the prepared baking sheet and stir with 1/2 teaspoon black pepper, 1 teaspoon salt, and 2 tablespoons oil. Roast the aubergine for 20 to 25 minutes, stirring halfway through, or until it is brown and soft.

•Once the red bell pepper has cooled down sufficiently, chop it into 1/4-inch pieces.

•Heat the remaining 2 tablespoons of olive oil in a medium Dutch oven over medium heat. Add the celery, onion, 1/2 teaspoon of black pepper, and the remaining 1 teaspoon of salt. Cook for 5 to 7 minutes, stirring often, or until golden. Add the bell pepper and eggplant and stir until thoroughly mixed. Cook the oregano and garlic together until aromatic.

3.ARTICHOKE DIP

Prep time: 10 minutes

Cook time: 30 minutes

Total time: 45 minutes

Serving: 8

Ingredients

- 2 cans (14 ounces each) artichoke hearts in water, rinsed, drained, and coarsely chopped
- 1⁄2 cup light mayonnaise
- 1⁄4 cup plus 1 tablespoon grated Parmesan cheese
- 1 tablespoon fresh lemon juice
- 1 garlic clove, coarsely chopped
- 1 scallion, minced, plus more for garnish
- Crudites (such as raw pepper wedges) or whole-wheat pita chips, for serving

Directions

•Set the oven's temperature to 425. Half the artichokes, the mayonnaise, 1/4 cup Parmesan, lemon juice, and garlic should all be placed in a food processor. Blend until silky.

•Once combined, pulse in the remaining artichokes and scallion. Spoon mixture into a baking dish that holds 1 quart. Add the last tablespoon of Parmesan on top.

•Bake for 30 to 35 minutes, or until bubbling and brown. Add some scallions as a garnish and serve with pita chips or crudites.

4.MEDITERRANEAN CROSTINI

Prep time: 15 minutes

Cook time: 10 minutes

Total time: 30 minutes

Serving: 4

Ingredients

- 1 can (15 1⁄2 ounces) chickpeas, drained and rinsed

- 1⁄4 cup plus 2 tablespoons extra-virgin olive oil

- 1 tablespoon freshly squeezed lemon juice

- 1 small garlic clove, minced

- Coarse salt and freshly ground pepper

- 8 large pitted green olives, cut into 1⁄8-inch slivers

- 2 tablespoons finely diced celery, plus celery leaves for garnish

- 12 slices (1⁄3 inch thick) baguette, toasted

Directions

•To make the spread, pulse the chickpeas, 1/4 cup oil, lemon juice, and garlic in a food processor. To make a smooth paste, pulse. Sprinkle with the salt and pepper, then reserve.

•Prepare relish: Olives, celery, and 1 tablespoon oil should all be combined in a small basin. Sprinkle with the salt and pepper, then reserve.

•Evenly distribute the chickpea spread among the toasts, then drizzle with olive relish. Add a drizzle of the leftover tablespoon of oil and season with pepper. Add celery leaves as a garnish and serve right away.

5.HOT SPINACH DIP

Prep time: 30 minutes

Cook time: 20 minutes

Total time: 1hour

Serving: 3 cups

Ingredients

- 2 teaspoons olive oil, plus more for baking dish

- 1 medium onion, diced

- 2 garlic cloves, minced

- 2 pounds spinach, cleaned, trimmed, and coarsely chopped

- 1/2 cup milk

- 6 ounces reduced-fat bar cream cheese

- 3 dashes Worcestershire sauce

- 3 dashes hot sauce, such as Tabasco

○ 3/4 cup shredded mozzarella

- Coarse salt and ground pepper

- Baguette slices, breadsticks, or crackers, for serving

Directions

•Set the oven's temperature to 425. Heat the oil in a big pot or Dutch oven over medium heat. Add the onion and garlic, and simmer for 5 to 8 minutes, or until lightly browned.

•Add the spinach in two batches, allowing it to wilt in between each addition; cook for 5 to 8 minutes, or until the spinach is thoroughly wilted. Move to a colander and squeeze to remove any surplus liquid before draining.

•Heat the milk in the same pot over high heat. Add cream cheese and whisk for three minutes or until melted. Stir together 1/4 cup mozzarella, spicy sauce, Worcestershire sauce, and spinach. Add pepper and salt for seasoning. Transfer into a shallow baking dish measuring 1 1/2 quarts, lightly oil it, and top with the leftover 1/2 cup of mozzarella. •Bake for 20 to 25 minutes, or until bubbling and golden brown. Serve warm.

6.WALNUT PATE

Prep time: 5 minutes

Cook time: 5 minutes

Total time: 4 hours 40 minutes Serving: 6

Ingredients

1 1/2 pounds fresh spinach (not baby), large stems removed 3/4 cup walnuts, plus more, chopped, for garnish

1/2 cup loosely packed fresh cilantro leaves

1/4 cup loosely packed fresh tarragon leaves

1/4 cup loosely packed fresh dill fronds 2 tablespoons white wine vinegar

3 scallions, roughly chopped

2 small cloves garlic, smashed

Kosher salt

1/4 teaspoon ground coriander Pinch cayenne pepper

2 tablespoons pomegranate seeds Crackers or crudites, for serving

Directions

•Special apparatus: 5 ramekins.

•Boil a big saucepan of water. Smooth out the plastic as much as you can into a 5-inch ramekin and line it with plastic wrap, allowing at least a 2-inch overhang.

•Add the spinach to the pot of water, toss to cover, and cook for about two minutes, or until wilted and soft. After draining, allow to cool fully. Remove as much water as possible from the spinach and cut it coarsely. Move to a medium-sized bowl.

•In a food processor, pulse together the walnuts, 1/3 cup warm water, dill, tarragon, cilantro, vinegar, scallions, garlic, 1 1/4 teaspoons salt, coriander, and cayenne until the mixture resembles mayonnaise.

Stir the spinach in the bowl with the walnut-herb combination.

7.GAZPACHO

Prep time: 20 minutes

Total time: 20 minutes

Serving: 5

Ingredients

1 hothouse cucumber, halved and seeded, but not peeled 2 red bell peppers, cored and seeded

4 plum tomatoes

1 red onion

3 garlic cloves, minced

23 ounces tomato juice (3 cups)

1/4 cup white wine vinegar

1/4 cup good olive oil

1/2 tablespoon kosher salt

1 teaspoons freshly ground black pepper

Directions

•Cut the tomatoes, red onions, bell peppers, and cucumbers into 1-inch cubes with a rough chop. Place every vegetable in a food processor with a steel blade and pulse until roughly chopped, each one at a time. Avoid overprocessing!

•Once all the vegetables have been pureed, put them in a big basin and mix in the olive oil, vinegar, tomato juice, garlic, salt, and pepper. Toss to combine, then chill to serve. The flavours of gazpacho intensify with time spent sitting.

8.WARM MARINATED OLIVES

Prep time: 20minutes

Total time: 20 minutes

Serving: 10

Ingredients

•2 cups large green olives with pits, such as Cerignola (11 ounces) 2 cups large black olives with pits, such as Kalamata (11 ounces) Zest of 1 orange, peeled in large strips

•4 large garlic cloves, smashed

•2 teaspoons whole fennel seeds

•2 teaspoons chopped fresh thyme leaves 3/4 teaspoon crushed red pepper flakes Kosher salt and freshly ground black pepper 2/3 cup good olive oil

•4 sprigs fresh thyme

Directions

•lAfter removing the black and green olives from their oil or brine, transfer them to a medium-sized bowl. Add the thyme leaves, orange zest, garlic, fennel seeds, red pepper flakes, 1/2 teaspoon each of salt and black pepper. Drizzle the blend with the extra virgin olive oil, toss in the thyme sprigs.

•Pour the mixture into a medium (10-inch) sauté pan, along with the olive oil. Simmer the oil over medium heat until it starts to crackle. Reduce the heat and sauté the garlic and olives for 4 to 5 minutes, stirring from time to time, or until aromatic and cooked through.

•Serve heated from out of the pan or transfer to a platter. Present a little dish to the pits

9.CLASSIC DEVILED EGGS

Prep time: 20 minutes

Cook time: 15 minutes

Total time: 35 minutes

Serving: 4

Ingredients

6 eggs

1/4 cup mayonnaise

1 teaspoon white vinegar

1 teaspoon yellow mustard

1/8 teaspoon salt

Freshly ground black pepper Smoked Spanish paprika, for garnish

Directions

•Put the eggs in a saucepan in a single layer and add enough water to cover the eggs by one and a half inches. After bringing the water to a boil on high, cover, reduce the heat, and let it cook for one minute. Take off the heat and cover for 14 minutes. After that, continually rinse under cold water for 1 minute.

•Egg shells should be cracked and gently peeled under cold running water. Dry with paper towels, being gentle. Cut the eggs in half lengthwise, then transfer the yolks to a medium-sized bowl while the whites are arranged on a tray for presenting. Using a fork, mash the yolks into a fine crumble. Mix thoroughly after adding the mustard, vinegar, mayonnaise, salt, and pepper.

•Distribute heaping teaspoons of the yolk mixture evenly..

10.TOASTED RAVIOLI

Prep time: 45 minutes

Cook time: 20 minutes

Total time:1 hour 5 minutes

Serving: 6

Ingredients

3/4 to 1 pound small fresh ravioli (meat and/or cheese) 3 large eggs, beaten

1 1/2 cups milk

2 cups breadcrumbs

3 tablespoons finely chopped fresh parsley 1 teaspoon finely chopped fresh rosemary Kosher salt and freshly ground pepper Vegetable oil, for frying

1/2 cup grated parmesan cheese Marinara sauce, for dipping

Directions

•Place the ravioli onto a baking sheet and freeze for 20 to 30 minutes, or until it becomes firm.

•In a pie plate or shallow dish, whisk together the milk and eggs. In another shallow dish, combine the breadcrumbs, parsley, rosemary, and 1/2 teaspoon of salt and pepper.

•Coat the ravioli in the breadcrumb mixture after dipping it in the egg mixture and allowing any excess to fall off. After about 15 minutes, return to the baking sheet and freeze until solid.

•In a deep skillet, heat up 1 inch of vegetable oil until a deep-fry thermometer reads 350 degrees Fahrenheit. Fry the ravioli in two or three batches for four to six minutes each, rotating as needed, until they are golden brown. After transferring to a baking sheet covered with paper towels to drain.

Chapter 2: Breakfast Delight

1.JAPANESE SOUFFLE PANCAKES

Prep time: 15 minutes

Cook time: 10 minutes

Total time: 25 minutes

Serving: 4

Ingredients

•21/2 tbsp skim milk

•6 tbsp cake flour

•1/4 tbsp vanilla extract

•1/4 tbsp cream of tartar

•1 tbsp unsalted butter

•1 tbsp baking powder

•3 tbsp granulated white sugar •Eggs (2-3)

•1/2 tbsp mayonnaise

Directions

•To combine the egg yolks, mayonnaise, baking powder, vanilla, and milk, use a medium-sized bowl. Using a flour sifter or fine mesh strainer, sift in cake flour (don't skip this step!). Whisk the batter until it's smooth and the mixture turns a light yellow colour.

•Combine sugar and cooled egg whites in the bowl of a stand mixer. Ensure that the whisk attachment and mixing bowl are dry and totally clean. The oil will prevent your egg whites from becoming meringue. Whip until stiff peaks form, using the fastest speed your mixer will allow. (Roughly two to three minutes) The meringue should be able to maintain its shape and should not slide when the mixing bowl is turned upside down.

2.EASY POTATO SKILLET

Prep time: 15 minutes

 Cook time: 45 minutes

Total time: 1hour

Serving:5

Ingredients

- 1and1⁄4 pounds russet potatoes, medium diced

- 1and1⁄4 pounds red potatoes, medium diced

- 1 of tablespoon canola oil

- 1 teaspoon cumin

- 1⁄2 teaspoon chilli powder

- 1⁄4 teaspoon salt

- 1 red bell pepper,diced

- 1 green bell pepper,diced

- 1 large yellow onion,diced

- 1 jalapeno,minced

- 3 cloves garlic,minced

- 1can(15.7ounce)black beans,drained and rinsed(about

1.5 cups)

- 1 bunch(12 ounces)spinach,stems removed

- 2 small avocados,for topping

- cilantro,for topping

Directions

● Setoventemperatureto425°F.Heatonetablespoonof canola oil in a sizable cast iron skillet or other oven-safe pan over medium heat. Add the salt, cumin, chilli powder, and diced potatoes once it's hot. Cook for only two minutes, stirring to coat evenly.

● For 20 Minutes,preheat the oven and place the cast-iron pan inside. Stir the pan halfway through.

● Addthebellpepper,onion,jalapenos,andgarlicafter20 minutes. Simmer for another fifteen minutes, stirring once. Return the cast iron to the stove after fifteen minutes.

● Onmediumheat,sautéthepotatoesuntiltheyarecooked through and have a light brown colour. Add the spinach and black beans and stir. When the spinach and black beans are fully heated, the skillet breakfast is ready.

3.BUCKWHEAT PORRIDGE

Prep time: 10 minutes

Cook time: 10 minutes

Total time: 20 minutes

Serving: 4

Ingredients

•1 cup roasted buckwheat groats

•3 cups water

•1 tablespoon unsalted butter(non-dairy for

vegans) optional •1/2 teaspoon salt

If Making Milk Porridge:

•1/2 cup plant-based milk

•1 teaspoon sweetener of choice optional

•fruit optional

Directions

● Heat water in a pot until it boils. Stir in raw buckwheat groats. Once the water has been absorbed, simmer the pot with a lid on for ten minutes. Once the heat is off, add the salt and leave it for a further ten minutes.

● Serve warm with a savoury dish topped with butter or as a porridge with milk and toppings.

4.PALEO MUESLI

Prep time: 5 minutes

Cook time: 20 minutes

Total time: 25 minutes

Serving: 12

Ingredients

•1 cup almonds {or any nuts of your choice} •1 cup cashews {or any nuts of your choice} •1/4 cup pumpkin seeds

•1/3 cup sunflower seeds

•1/3 cup coconut oil

•1/3 cup pure maple syrup

•1 tbsp cinnamon

•2 tsp pure vanilla extract

•1/3 cup unsweetened shredded coconut •1 tsp sea salt

•1/4 cup hemp hearts

•1 cup freeze dried strawberries

Directions

•Set oven temperature to 325°F.

•In a food processor, pulse the nuts, pumpkin seeds, and sunflower seeds until a pleasant mixture of small and large bits forms. Pro tip: not using a food processor? Using a sharp knife, chop the nuts.

1/4 cup pumpkin seeds, 1/3 cup sunflower seeds, and 1 cup cashews •Mix the coconut oil, maple syrup, cinnamon, and vanilla in a microwave-safe bowl. The coconut oil should melt in the microwave in 30 seconds.

1 tablespoon cinnamon, 2 teaspoons pure vanilla essence, 1/3 cup coconut oil, and 1/3 cup pure maple syrup

•Stir together the chopped nuts and seeds, coconut oil mixture, and remaining ingredients (strawberries excluded).

1/4 cup hemp hearts, 1/3 cup unsweetened shredded coconut, and 1 tsp sea salt

5.INDONESIAN BLACK RICE PUDDING

Prep time: 5 minutes

Cook time: 1hour

Total time: 1 hour 5 minutes Serving: 4

INGREDIENTS

- 1 cup of Indonesian black rice

- 14 oz can full-fat coconut milk

- 1 1/2 cups water *reduce to 1 cup for Instant Pot

- a pinch of salt

- 2 tablespoon coconut sugar or other sweetener (see notes)

- diced banana, coconut chips, and hemp hearts for garnish

Direction

TO MAKE ON THE STOVE TOP

•Place the black rice, 1 1/2 cups water, salt, and coconut milk (save a couple of tablespoons for drizzling, if preferred) in a medium-sized pot.

•Once the rice is soft and most of the liquid has been absorbed, bring to a boil, lower the heat and simmer covered. You want to leave some liquid behind because the pudding will continue to thicken as it cools. This will take approximately one hour, so periodically check on the cooking process and give it a thorough stir.

•After the rice has finished cooking, turn off the heat and whisk in one tablespoon of your preferred sweetener. Then, taste. You might decide not to include another.

6.EGG IN A SQUASH HOLE

Prep time: 5 minutes

 Cook time: 30 minutes

Total time: 35 minutes

Serving: 2

INGREDIENTS

- 4 rings winter squash eg butternut or acorn

- 4 large eggs

- 2 teaspoons extra virgin olive oil

- salt and pepper

Directions

•Set oven temperature to 200°C/400°F.

•Line baking sheet with parchment paper.

•Saute the squash rings in a little olive oil, then season with salt and pepper. Place in a single layer on the baking sheet that has been preheated.

 •Squash rings should be baked for ten minutes. They should be fork-tender but not soft at this point.

•After taking the squash out of the oven, carefully turn them over with a spatula. Apply a thin layer of olive oil on the parchment paper centred within the squash rings.

•Carefully slip one cracked egg into the centre of a squash ring from a small bowl. Continue with the remaining eggs.

•After the egg white is set and the yolk has just a hint of colour, place the tray in the oven and bake for 12 minutes.

7.SPELT FLOUR PANCAKES

Prep time: 10 minutes

Cook time: 20 minutes

Total time: 30 minutes

Serving: 12

INGREDIENTS

- 3 Tablespoons melted butter, and slightly cooled

- 1 cup plain full-fat yoghourt

- 2 large eggs

- 2 teaspoons vanilla extract

- 3⁄4 cup wholegrain spelt flour

- 1⁄2 cup all purpose flour

- 2 Tablespoons granulated sugar

- 2 teaspoons baking powder

- 1⁄2 teaspoons salt

- 1⁄4 cup milk if needed

- butter for the pan

Directions

- Melt the butter and leave it to cool.Butter, three tablespoons

- Combine yoghurt, eggs, melted butter, and vanilla essence in a big bowl.

- Two large eggs, one cup plain full-fat yoghurt, and two tablespoons vanilla

extract

- Add the spelt flour, all-purpose flour, baking powder, sugar, and salt to the same bowl.

● 2 Tablespoons granulated sugar, 2 teaspoons baking powder, 1/2 teaspoon salt, and 3/4 cup wholegrain spelt wheat combined with 1/2 cup all-purpose flour

● Using a fork or spatula, gently stir the dry ingredients on top of the wet mix until the wet and dry ingredients are combined.

● Gradually add milk until your pancake batter reaches the right consistency.

● 1/2 cup of milk

● Over medium-high heat, preheat a big cast-iron skillet or heavy-based nonstick pan.

8.NON-SUGAR BANANA BRAN MUFFINS

Prep time: 30 minutes

Cook time: 25 minutes

Total time: 55 minutes

Serving: 12

INGREDIENTS

- 1 1/2 cups chopped pitted dates about 200g dates

- 1 cup water

- 1 teaspoon baking soda

- 2 large very ripe bananas mashed

- 3 Tablespoons of soft butter OR neutral-flavoured oil I've used both with the same results

- 2 large eggs

- 1 cup milk regular milk or plant-based milk both work fine

- 1 1/2 cups wheat bran

- 1/2 cup of rolled oats

- 2 cups whole wheat flour

- 1 Tablespoon baking powder

- 1/2 teaspoon salt

- 1 banana diced

- 1 cup walnuts chopped

Directions

•Preheat the oven to 200°C/400°F and grease your muffin pans (I use butter for this).

•Place the dates and water in a small (but not too small!) pot and bring to a boil over high heat. As soon as the water boils, add the baking soda and whisk to mix. Be •amazed by the science of foam and don't worry about spilling any; just make sure your pot is big enough to prevent foaming over. Remove mixture and let it cool.

•One cup water, one 1⁄2 cups chopped pitted dates, and one teaspoon baking soda

•Mash bananas and butter or olive oil should be combined in a stand mixer until the mixture is light and foamy.

•Three tablespoons of soft butter OR neutral-flavoured oil, two large, extremely ripe bananas.

9.MAPLE APPLE GRANOLA

Prep time: 10

Cook time: 30

Total time: 40

Serving: 12

INGREDIENTS

- 3⁄4 cup unsweetened applesauce

- 1⁄2 cup good quality maple syrup

- 1⁄3 cup extra virgin olive oil

- 5 cups rolled oats

- 1 cup walnut pieces chopped

- 1 teaspoon coarse sea salt

- 1 teaspoon ground cinnamon

Directions

•Preheat the oven to 325°F, or 160°C. Put parchment paper between two baking pans and mix the applesauce, maple syrup, and olive oil together in a large dish.

•Add the oats, walnut pieces, cinnamon, and salt and stir. Completely mix.

•On the two preheated baking sheets, distribute the mixture equally.

•Place the baking sheets in the upper and lower thirds of the oven and bake for ten minutes. Remove from the oven, lift the edges of the parchment paper so the granola falls into the centre of the pan, and mix in the cereal. Place the granola back in the oven after flipping the pans over.

•Bake for a further 10 minutes, then stir the granola and flip the pans over again.

•Bake for a further ten minutes.

10.RICOTTA AND SPINACH EGG BAKE

Prep time: 5 minutes

Cook time: 15 minutes

Total time: 20 minutes

 Serving: 1

INGREDIENTS

- butter for greasing the ramekin

- 1/4 cup ricotta cheese

- 1/2 cup roughly chopped spinach

- 1/2 teaspoon dried thyme

- 1/2 teaspoon lemon zest optional

- 1 tablespoon olive oil

- 2 eggs

- salt and pepper

- 2 slices bread for serving

Directions

- Set the oven temperature to 375°F (195°C).

- Grease a small baking dish or ramekin.

- Combine the ricotta, spinach, thyme, lemon zest, olive oil, and a small pinch

of salt and pepper in a small bowl.

- After lining the ramekin with the ricotta mixture, make two tiny wells to hold

the eggs.

- Pour two eggs into each ramekin, cover with a little olive oil, and bake.

- Bake for 12 to 15 minutes, or until the yolks are still somewhat runny but the whites are set.

- Take out of the oven and pair with warm buttered bread.

Chapter 3: Luscious Lunches

1.SPICY KEDGEREE

Prep time: 10 minutes
Cook time: 1hour
Total time: 1 hour 10 minutes
Serving: 4

Ingredients

- 350g long grain brown rice
- 150g green beans, trimmed and halved
- 4 medium eggs
- 2 tbsp olive oil
- 2 sliced onions
- 2 garlic cloves, crushed
- 2 heaped tbsp medium curry powder
- 1 tsp ground turmeric
- 2 bay leaves
- 200g spinach
- 100g cherry tomatoes, halved
- 1/2 small bunch coriander, chopped
- 1 green chilli, sliced
- 1 lemon, cut into wedges

Directions

Step 1: Run cold water over the rice and rub it with your fingers to get rid of extra starch. Cook as directed on the package, then make sure to drain well.

Step 2: Simmer a second pan of water. After cooking the green beans for two minutes, use a slotted spoon to transfer them to a bowl and put them aside. After 7 minutes of boiling in the pan, remove the eggs and place them in a bowl of cold water to cool.

Step 3: In the interim, warm up the oil in a sizable skillet over medium heat. Fry the onions until golden, ten to fifteen minutes. Cook for a further minute after adding the bay leaves, curry powder, turmeric, and garlic. Cook after adding the tomatoes, spinach, and a little water.

2.CAVOLO NERO ORECCHIETTE

Prep time: 10 minutes
 Cook time: 20 minutes
Total time: 30 minutes
Serving: 2

Ingredients

- 150 g orecchiette
- 200g cavolo nero, separated into stems and leaves
- 1 tbsp olive oil
- 3 garlic cloves, crushed
- 1 red chilli (deseeded if you like), finely chopped
- 1 banana shallot, finely chopped
- 1 lemon, zested and juiced
- 75g ricotta
- 15g almonds, roughly chopped and toasted

Directions

STEP 1: Cook the orecchiette according to the directions on the package, then drain, setting aside a large mug of water. Chop the cavolo nero leaves and stems finely, being careful to keep them apart. In a large skillet, heat the olive oil and sauté the stems, garlic, shallot, and chilli for five minutes over low heat, until the vegetables are tender. Next, add the cavolo nero leaves and stir. Add the pasta and toss to mix after you have fried it until it's barely wilted.

Step 2: Add the ricotta, lemon zest, and juice, and season with a little splash of the pasta water that was set aside. To serve, scatter the almonds on top.

3.GIANT BUTTER BEAN STEW

Prep time: 30 minutes
Cook time: 1 hour 15 minutes
Total time: 1 hour 45 minutes
Serving: 6

Ingredients

- 4 x 235g cans butter beans or 500g dried butter beans (cook according to pack instructions)
- 100ml Greek extra virgin olive oil
- 3 small red onions, finely sliced
- 2 large carrots, finely sliced
- 3 celery stalks with leaves, finely chopped
- 4 sundried tomatoes, sliced
- 1kg ripe tomatoes, skinned, deseeded and finely chopped
- 4 garlic cloves, chopped
- 1 tsp paprika
- 1 tsp ground cinnamon
- 2 tbsp tomato purée
- 1 tsp sugar
- small pack flat-leaf parsley, finely chopped
- small pack dill, finely chopped
- 100g feta (optional), crumbled

Directions

Step 1: Pour the beans from the can, setting aside 200ml of the liquid. In a large casserole dish with a lid that is flameproof, heat the oil and saute the onions, carrots, and celery until they are soft and transparent, but not browned. Stir in the other ingredients, save half of the feta (if using) and chopped herbs.

Step 2: Preheat the oven to 180°C (160°C for fans) or gas 4. After 5 more minutes of moderate cooking, pour the conserved liquid on top. Bake the dish for 40 minutes with a cover on. Periodically make sure the beans are not drying out; if necessary, add a bit more water.

Step 3: Take off the lid and continue baking for an additional ten minutes. Reheat after two days of preparation.

4.CREAMY TOMATO RISOTTO

Prep time: 5 minutes
Cook time: 35 minutes
Total time: 40 minutes
Serving: 4

Ingredients

- 400g can chopped tomato
- 1l vegetable stock
- knob of butter
- 1 tbsp olive oil
- 1 onion, finely chopped
- 2 garlic cloves, finely chopped
- 1 rosemary sprig, finely chopped

- 250g risotto rice
- 300g cherry tomato, halved
- small pack basil, roughly torn
- 4 tbsp grated parmesan

Directions

STEP 1: Put half of the stock and the diced tomatoes in a food processor; pulse until smooth. Transfer into a saucepan with the leftover stock, heat gently, and maintain over low heat.

STEP 2: In the meantime, put the oil and butter in the bottom of a big saucepan and heat it slowly until the butter melts. When the onion is tender, add it and simmer it gently for 6 to 8 minutes. Saute the garlic and rosemary for one more minute after adding them. Stir the rice in and simmer for one minute.

Step 3: About a quarter at a time, begin adding the heated stock and tomato mixture. As the stock is absorbed, add additional and continue to toss the risotto while cooking. Once you've included

Step 4: After a minute, uncover and mix in the basil. Add some Parmesan cheese and freshly ground pepper as garnish.

5.CHILLI CORNBREAD PIE

Prep time: 20 minutes
Cook time: 50 minutes
Total time: 1 hour 10 minutes
Serving: 4

Instagram

- 2 tsp rapeseed oil
- 2 red onions (320g), finely chopped
- 2 celery sticks (about 150g), sliced
- 1 tbsp hot chilli powder
- 1 tbsp ground coriander
- 1 tsp ground cumin
- 3 garlic cloves, finely grated
- 500g carton passata
- 2 x 400g cans three bean salad in water
- 2 tsp gluten-free vegetable bouillon powder
- 20g coriander, leaves picked and chopped

Directions

- STEP 1: In a nonstick pan set over medium heat, heat the oil and cook the onions and celery for 8 minutes, turning frequently. Add the garlic and spices, then pour in the

 passata, bean salad (with the can contents included), and bouillon. After ten minutes of simmering under cover, mix in the coriander. Spoon onto a small, oven-safe dish and allow it to cool down a little.
- Step 2: Preheat the oven to 190°C (or 170°C with a fan) or gas 5. Place the gramme flour, baking powder, chilli powder, and cornmeal in a bowl and well combine. In a separate bowl, beat the egg, yoghurt, and milk together. Pour the mixture into the dry ingredients and stir to form a batter. Pour the cheese mixture over the bean after stirring it in.

6.HALLOUMI PASTA

Prep time: 15 minutes
Cook time: 25 minutes
Total time: 40 minutes
Serving: 4

Ingredients

- 250g wholemeal penne
- 1 tsp rapeseed oil

- 120g halloumi, halved through the seam and cut into cubes
- 325g baby plum tomatoes on the vine, halved
- 320g courgettes, cut into cubes
- 3 garlic cloves, finely grated
- 400g can chopped tomatoes
- 6 pitted Kalamata olives, quartered
- 1 tsp dried oregano
- 10g parsley, chopped

Directions

- Step 1: Cook the pasta as directed on the packet. As this is going on, heat the oil in a sizable, deep, nonstick skillet over medium heat and cook the halloumi for three minutes, tossing regularly, until it browns. Transfer to a platter and allow the tomatoes to soften in the pan for one to two minutes. Pour into the halloumi bowl.

- Step 2: Add the tinned tomatoes, whisk in the oregano and olives, and toss in the courgettes and garlic after a quick stir-fry. Simmer, covered, for ten minutes.

- Step 3: Drain the pasta and combine it with the sauce, baby plum tomatoes, halloumi, and parsley. Serve half at once and save the other half for a later time. Will store for up to 3 days, covered and refrigerated.

7.EGG-FRIED NOODLES WITH BEANSPROUTS

Prep time: 10 minutes
Cook time: 12 minutes
 Total time: 22 minutes
Serving: 2

Ingredients

- 2 dried wholemeal noodle nests (about 100g)
- 2 limes, juiced
- 1 tsp tamari
- 2 garlic cloves, 1 finely grated, 1 chopped
- 1 red chilli, deseeded and finely sliced
- 1 tbsp sesame or rapeseed oil
- 2 red onions, (200g), halved and thinly sliced
- 15g ginger, peeled and cut into fine shreds
- 1 small red pepper, deseeded and cut into strips
- 1 tbsp medium curry powder
- 200g ready-to-eat beansprouts, rinsed and drained
- 1 tbsp tahini
- 3 eggs, beaten
- 15g coriander, chopped

Directions

STEP 1: Cook the noodles as directed on the package. In a small bowl, mix together the lime juice, tamari, grated garlic, and chilli. Put aside.

STEP 2: Heat the oil in a large, wide skillet or nonstick wok over high heat. Stir-fry the onions, ginger, and pepper for 5 minutes, or until they are tender. In the final minute, add the chopped garlic. After adding the curry powder, simmer for an additional minute. After adding the beansprouts, sauté them until they are hot and beginning to soften. Stir in the tahini.

STEP 3: Push the vegetables to one side of the wok and add the egg; a little extra oil may be needed. After the eggs have mostly set, stir-fry them.

8.ARTICHOKE AND AUBERGINE RICE

Prep time: 15 minutes
Cook time: 50 minutes
 Total time: 1hour 5 minutes
Serving: 6

Ingredients

- 60ml olive oil
- 2 aubergines, cut into chunks
- 1 large onion, finely chopped
- 2 garlic cloves, crushed
- small pack parsley, leaves picked, stalks finely chopped
- 2 tsp smoked paprika
- 2 tsp turmeric
- 400g paella rice
- 1 1/2l vegetable stock
- 2 x 175g packs chargrilled artichokes
- 2 lemons 1 juiced, 1 cut into wedges to serve

Directions

STEP 1: In a large nonstick frying pan or paella pan, heat 2 tablespoons of oil. Remove and set aside the aubergines after they are beautifully coloured on all sides (you can add another tablespoon of oil if they start to catch too much). When the onion is softened, add another tablespoon of oil to the pan and sauté it gently for two to three minutes. After a few more minutes of cooking the garlic and parsley stems, add the rice and spices and stir until everything is well coated. After two minutes of heating, add half of the stock and cook, uncovered, over medium heat for twenty minutes, stirring now and again to keep from sticking.

Step 2: Gently fold in the artichokes and aubergine and cover the remaining portion.

9.VEGGIE NUGGETS WITH SUMMER SLAW

Prep time: 35 minutes
Cook time: 40 minutes
Total time: 1hour 15 minutes
Serving: 4

Ingredients

- 100g quinoa
- 2 onions (320g), very finely chopped
- 2 tbsp olive oil, plus 1 tbsp for cooking the next day
- 2 x 400g cans black beans, drained
- 2 tsp dried oregano
- 31⁄2 tbsp crunchy peanut butter
- 3 tbsp parsley, chopped
- 1 tsp vegetable bouillon powder
- 2 eggs, beaten

For the coleslaw

- 90g pot bio yogurt
- 1 tsp English mustard powder
- 1 tsp apple cider vinegar
- 1 carrot (150g), coarsely grated
- 1 red pepper, deseeded and finely chopped
- 1 very small onion, finely chopped
- 320g white cabbage, finely shredded
- 4 tbsp chopped coriander

Directions

STEP 1: Cook the quinoa for 20 minutes, as directed on the package, then let it stand for 5 minutes before thoroughly draining. As this is going on, sauté the onions in 1 tablespoon oil over medium-low heat for 5 minutes with the lid on, then remove and continue to sauté for a further 5 minutes, or until they are soft and beginning to turn colour. Turn off the heat and add the black beans, parsley, peanut butter, oregano, and bouillon. Mash everything with a potato masher until the beans are crushed. Gently stir in the eggs and quinoa.

STEP 2: Heat the remaining tablespoon of oil in a big, nonstick frying pan. Then, add rounded spoonfuls of the mixture to the pan, spacing them apart, using a measuring tablespoon. Cook for approximately 3 minutes.

STEP 3: To prepare the cole slaw, combine the yoghurt, vinegar, and mustard powder in a bowl. Whisk to create a dressing. Add the veggies and coriander and mix again. Present two portions of the nuggets along with half of the coleslaw. The rest can be refrigerated for up to three days.

10.GREEN GODDESS SALAD

Prep time: 20 minutes
Serving: 10

Ingredients

- 2 heads fennel, finely shaved
- 4 Baby Gem lettuces, cut into wedges
- 1 cucumber, cut into finger-size batons

- 1 bunch spring onion, cut into finger-size batons For the dressing
- 1 tbsp Dijon mustard
- 2 tbsp red wine vinegar
- 6 tbsp olive oil

Directions

Step 1: Pour the components for the dressing into a jar, add a little water, and give it a good shake.

Step 2: Transfer the salad to a bowl and refrigerate for a maximum of 24 hours. Decorate the salad before serving.

Chapter 4: Delectable Dinners

1.BRAISED SESAME TOFU

Prep time: 10 minutes
Cook time: 15 minutes
Serving: 2

Ingredients

- 400g extra-firm tofu
- 1⁄2 tbsp reduced-salt soy sauce
- 1 tbsp mirin
- 1⁄2 tbsp gochujang
- 3 garlic cloves, finely chopped
- 2 tsp sesame seeds
- 2 spring onions, finely sliced
- 1 tbsp rapeseed oil
- 200g green beans
- cooked brown rice, to serve

Directions

Step 1: Pat the block of tofu dry, then cut it in half lengthwise, then into slices that are one centimetre thick. While preparing the braise, place it aside on a plate lined with kitchen paper and weigh it down with another sheet of paper and plate on top. Combine the soy sauce with the 200ml of water, the gochujang, garlic, sesame seeds, and the majority of the spring onions.

Step 2: Heat the oil in a pan over medium-high heat and cook the tofu until golden brown, 4–5 minutes per side. After adding the soy sauce mixture, distribute the green beans evenly. After bringing to a simmer, cook the green beans over medium heat for ten minutes, or until the braising liquid has thickened.

Step 3: Garnish with the leftover spring onions and accompany the dish with brown rice.

2.CURRIED SATAY NOODLES

prep time: 15 minutes
Cook time: 20 minutes
Serving: 2

Ingredients

- 150g dried wholewheat noodles
- 2 tsp rapeseed oil
- 1 red pepper, halved seeded and thinly sliced
- 1 carrot, cut into matchsticks (about 90g)
- 1 tbsp finely chopped ginger

- 3 garlic cloves, finely chopped
- 1 chilli, deseeded and finely chopped (optional)
- 1/2 tsp cumin seeds
- 1-2 tsp curry powder
- 2 1/2 -3 tbsp crunchy peanut butter
- 1 tbsp tomato purée
- 150ml vegetable stock, made with 1/2 tsp vegetable bouillon
- 100g frozen peas
- 1/2 lemon, juiced

Directions

STEP 1: Boil the noodles as directed on the package, then make sure the strands are separated by giving them a thorough rinse. In the meantime, stir-fry the pepper, carrot, ginger, garlic, and chilli, if using, for 5 minutes or until they are softened. In a wok or sauté pan, heat oil over high heat. Add the curry powder and cumin seeds, and heat for about 30 seconds, or until aromatic.

STEP 2: Using the vegetable stock, blend the peanut butter and tomato purée until smooth. After adding the frozen peas and the drained noodles to the wok, add the tomato and peanut sauce and stir everything together. Add a drop extra water and stir if it appears a little claggy. Add the lemon juice, stir it very well, and then serve.

3.VEGETABLE BAKE

Prep time: 20 minutes
 Cook time: 1hour
Serving: 6-8

Ingredients

- 1 celeriac, peeled and cut into cubes (about 950g)
- 1 cauliflower, broken into florets, stem finely chopped, leaves reserved
- 3 garlic cloves, unpeeled and bashed
- 2 tsp maple syrup
- 2 tbsp olive oil
- 2 leeks, halved and finely sliced
- 350g chestnut mushrooms, sliced
- small handful of thyme sprigs
- 200ml dry white wine
- 50g unsalted butter
- 50g plain flour
- 700ml whole milk
- 100g extra-mature cheddar, grated
- 100g sourdough, blitzed to breadcrumbs

Directions

Step 1: Preheat the oven to 200°C (180°C for fans or gas). 6. In a roasting tin, toss together the celeriac, cauliflower florets and stems, garlic, and maple syrup with 1 tablespoon olive oil. Season to taste. Bake for 30 to 35 minutes, or until the vegetables are caramelised. Take out of the oven, scoop out the roasted garlic cloves, and use a fork to mash them on a cutting board before setting them aside. Transfer the remaining roasted vegetable mixture to a baking dish.

STEP 2: In the meantime, sauté the leeks, mushrooms, and thyme sprigs in a large frying pan with the remaining oil over medium-low heat for ten to fifteen minutes, or until the vegetables are tender. For five minutes, turn the heat up just a little bit to caramelise the leeks and mushrooms.

Step 3: Cook the wine until it has reduced almost all. Once the butter starts to foam, stir in the flour. Cook, stirring, for a few minutes. Add the milk little by little, stirring thoroughly after each addition. Bring to a low simmer and boil, stirring frequently, until thickened, 5 minutes. Take off the heat, then add the cheddar and the mashed roasted garlic, stirring until the cheese melts. Properly season. Chop the cauliflower leaves coarsely and mix them into the sauce.

Step 4: Add the cheese sauce and roasted vegetables to the baking dish, stirring to mix. After adding the sourdough crumbs, bake for a further 15 to 20 minutes, or until the sauce is bubbling and the top is brown.

4.SWEET POTATO AND PEANUT CURRY

Prep time: 15 minutes
Cook time: 45 minutes
Serving: 4

Ingredients

- 1 tbsp coconut oil
- 1 onion, chopped
- 2 garlic cloves, grated
- thumb-sized piece ginger, grated
- 3 tbsp Thai red curry paste (check the label to make sure it's vegetarian/ vegan)
- 1 tbsp smooth peanut butter
- 500g sweet potato, peeled and cut into chunks
- 400ml can coconut milk
- 200g bag spinach
- 1 lime, juiced
- cooked rice, to serve (optional)
- dry roasted peanuts, to serve (optional)

Directions

Step 1: In a saucepan over medium heat, melt 1 tablespoon coconut oil and cook 1 chopped onion for 5 minutes. Add a thumb-sized piece of grated ginger and two grated garlic cloves, and simmer for one minute, or until fragrant.

STEP 2: Stir in 500g of peeled and chopped sweet potatoes, 1 tablespoon smooth peanut butter, and 3 tablespoons Thai red curry paste. Finally, add 200ml of water and 400ml of coconut milk.

STEP 3 Bring to a boil, reduce the heat, and simmer, uncovered, until the sweet potato is tender, 25 to 30 minutes.

STEP 4: Stir in 200g spinach and 1 lime juice; season to taste. Serve with cooked rice and top with a handful of dry-roasted peanuts for crunch.

5.CHEESE AND CARAMELISED ONION TART

Prep time: 40 minutes
Cook time: 2hours
Serving: 8-10

Ingredients

- 50g butter
- 800g onions (about 8), finely sliced
- 300ml double cream
- small pinch of grated nutmeg
- 4 egg yolks (freeze the whites for another recipe, such as meringue)
- 100g mature vegetarian cheddar, grated, plus extra to serve
(optional)
- chives, finely sliced, to serve
For the pastry
- 200g plain flour, plus extra for dusting
- 125g cold butter, cut into cubes
- 1 egg, beaten

Directions

Step 1: Prepare the pastry first. Place the flour and butter in a bowl and use your fingertips to press the ingredients together until they resemble coarse breadcrumbs. Add the egg and use your hands to mix everything until it's just blended. Become a disc in shape. Will freeze for up to a month or store covered and refrigerated for up to two days.

STEP 2: Using a surface dusted with flour, roll out the pastry to form a disc about 28 cm in diameter. Lift it over a 23cm tart tin with the rolling pin and wrap it over the tin. Leaving the excess dough to overhang, use a small ball made of leftover pastry scraps to press the pastry into the tin's base and up its side. Relax

STEP 3: In the meantime, melt the butter in a skillet over low to medium heat and sauté the onions for 45 minutes, turning periodically and sprinkling heavily with salt, until they get brown and sticky. After adding the cream, whisk in the nutmeg. After bringing to a simmer, turn the heat off.

Step 4: Preheat the oven to 200°C (180°C with a fan) or gas 6. Using a fork, lightly pierce the entire base of the tart. Next, cover with a big circle of baking paper and stuff with dried rice, pulses, or baking beans. Bake for another 10 to 15 minutes, or until light brown, after removing the paper and beans after 20 minutes of baking. To make sure it's done, break off a small piece of the pastry that is hanging over.

Step 5: In the meantime, beat in the egg yolks and two-thirds of the cheese to the onion and cream mixture. Pour into the pastry case, top with the remaining cheese, and bake for 20 to 25 minutes, or until the cheese is golden and set. Allow it to cool fully in the pan, then use a serrated knife to trim the excess before removing it from the pan. If desired, top with additional cheese and chives. Leftovers can be refrigerated for up to two days. To serve, reheat in a low oven.

6.CHILLI PANEER

Prep time: 20 minutes
Cook time: 20 minutes
Serving: 2

Ingredients

- 4 tbsp vegetable oil
- 2 tbsp cornflour
- 2 tbsp plain flour
- 1/2 tsp Kashmiri chilli powder
- 226g paneer, cut into 1cm cubes
- 1 spring onion, finely sliced
- cooked rice, to serve For the sauce
- 2 tsp cornflour
- 1 tbsp dark soy sauce
- 11/2-2 tbsp hot chilli sauce, to taste
- 11/2 tbsp ketchup
- 1 tsp rice vinegar
- 1 tsp honey
- 25g ginger, peeled and finely grated
- 4 garlic cloves, crushed
- 1 green chilli, finely chopped (deseeded if you like)
- 1/2 tsp Kashmiri chilli powder
- 1 red onion, roughly chopped
- 1 green pepper, deseeded and roughly chopped

Directions

STEP 1: In a sizable nonstick pan, warm the vegetable oil over medium heat. In a bowl, mix together the cornflour, plain flour, chilli powder, 1 tsp fine sea salt, 1/2 tsp freshly crushed black pepper, and 2 tbsp water to form a smooth paste. If the paste seems too thick, add a little more water to thin it out. Toss to coat after adding the paneer cubes. The coated paneer should be carefully tipped into the heated oil in the pan and cooked, stirring, until it is crisp and browned all over. Place on a kitchen paper-lined platter and reserve.

STEP 2: To prepare the sauce, pour the soy sauce into a jug with the cornflour and stir slowly to combine. Add the rice, ketchup, and chilli sauce. Whisk in the vinegar, honey, and 90 millilitres of water, then leave aside. Once the excess oil has been mostly drained from the pan, heat it back to medium. Add the chopped chilli, garlic, and ginger and fry for a few minutes until fragrant. Increase the heat to medium-high and add the pepper, onion, and chilli powder. Fry until

gently browned. Pour in the bubbling soy sauce mixture and let it thicken slightly.

Step 3: Turn off the heat and add the paneer, stirring to coat it thoroughly in the sauce. If necessary, add a little extra water, and adjust the seasoning. If desired, top with rice and sprinkle with the spring onions.

7.GINGERY BROCCOLI-FRY WITH CASHEW

Prep time: 15 minutes
Cook time: 10 minutes
Serving: 2

Ingredients

- 320g head of broccoli, stalks and florets separated
- 40g cashews, roughly chopped
- 1 tbsp sesame oil
- 15g ginger, finely sliced
- 1 small red onion, finely chopped
- 1 red pepper, deseeded and cut into thin strips
- 1 large carrot (160g), cut into thin strips
- 2 garlic cloves, thinly sliced
- 1 red chilli, deseeded and finely chopped, plus extra sliced, to serve
- 1 tbsp tamari
- 1 lime, juiced and zested
- 7g chopped coriander, plus extra to serve
- 2 eggs, beaten

Directions

Step 1: Finely chop the broccoli stems in a food processor. To make the texture resemble rice, add the florets and pulse one more.

Step 2: In a wok or frying pan, lightly brown the cashews. Transfer to a plate and reserve. Add the ginger, onion, pepper, carrot, garlic, and chilli to a skillet of heated oil over high heat. Stir-fry until beginning to brown, 2 to 3 minutes; cover and continue cooking for an additional 2 minutes.

Step 3: Stir-fry the broccoli with 3 tablespoons water for 3 minutes, or until all the vegetables are soft. Stir thoroughly after adding the tamari, lime juice, zest, and coriander. Next, add the eggs and quickly stir-fry them.

8.SIMPLE MUSHROOM CURRY

Prep time: 15 minutes
Cook time: 35 minutes
Serving: 4

Ingredients

- 50g unsalted butter
- 500g chestnut mushrooms, quartered
- 4-6 tbsp sunflower oil
- 1 tsp cumin seeds
- 1 tsp fennel seeds
- 1 large onion, finely chopped
- 4 garlic cloves, finely chopped
- 1 tsp ground ginger
- 1/4 tsp ground turmeric
- 1/2 tsp Kashmiri chilli powder
- 1/2 tsp garam masala
- 400g can chopped tomatoes
- 1 tsp caster sugar
- 2 tbsp thick, full-fat Greek yogurt
- 2 tbsp chopped coriander
- cooked rice or naan, to serve

Directions

- STEP1

Melt the butter in a large wok, karahi or non-stick frying pan over a medium-high heat and cook the mushrooms for 10 mins, or until any moisture has evaporated and they're starting to brown. Transfer to a bowl and set aside.

- STEP2

Heat the oil in the same pan over a medium-high heat and fry the cumin and fennel seeds, stirring continuously for about 30 seconds until they release a nutty aroma. Stir in the onion and cook for 12-15 mins until golden. Reduce the heat to medium, then add the garlic and continue frying for 1 min. Add the ginger, turmeric, chilli powder and garam masala, followed by the tomatoes and sugar. Cook, uncovered, for 5-7 mins, or until the masala thickens and a layer of oil forms around the edge of the pan.

- STEP3

Spoon the yogurt into a small bowl, add a small ladleful of the hot masala and mix well before stirring the yogurt into the pan of masala. Pour in 100ml hot water and simmer for 3-4 mins until the curry has the consistency of double cream. Season to taste, then return the mushrooms to the pan and stir to warm through. Scatter with the chopped coriander and serve with boiled rice or naan, if you like.

9.ROAST GARLIC AND TAHINI SPINACH

Prep time: 5 minutes
Cook time: 50 minutes
Serving: 6

Ingredients

- olive oil, for drizzling
- 1 whole garlic bulb
- 4 tbsp tahini
- 750g spinach, any thick stems removed and larger leaves chopped

Directions

Step 1: Season the garlic bulb with 1/2 tsp salt and drizzle with a little olive oil. Place the foil-wrapped item on the grill near the heat source, but away from the flames. Simmer for 35 to 40 minutes or until tender, then remove and let cool until manageable.

Step 2: Squeeze out half of the roasted garlic and mash it with a fork to form a paste. Add the tahini, 1/2 teaspoon sugar, 1/2 teaspoon salt, and 1/2 teaspoon black pepper, and thoroughly mix. Add 4–5 tablespoons of water, or just enough to create a light, loose dressing.

Step 3: Place a flameproof pan directly over the embers on the grill and cook the spinach for a few minutes, stirring occasionally, until it wilts and becomes soft.

10.TOFU STIR-FRY

Prep time: 15
 Cook time: 15
Serving: 4

Ingredients

- 3 tbsp low-sodium soy sauce
- 11/2 tbsp honey
- 1 tbsp white wine vinegar
- 300g tofu, cut into chunks
- 2 tbsp sunflower oil
- 2 garlic cloves, sliced
- 2cm piece ginger, sliced
- 2 carrots, sliced into thin batons
- 300g broccoli, cut into small florets
- 1 red pepper, sliced into strips
- 1 tsp cornflour

To garnish

- 1 spring onion, sliced
- 2 tsp sesame seeds
- small bunch of coriander, chopped

Directions

Step 1: Combine the vinegar, honey, and soy sauce in a bowl and set it aside.

Step 2: Pat the tofu chunks dry and generously season. In a large frying pan, heat half the oil over high heat. Fry the tofu for 5 minutes, stirring periodically, until golden. Fry the ginger and garlic together for a further minute. Spoon half of the soy dressing over the tofu mixture in a bowl and set aside.

Step 3: Fill the wok with the leftover oil. When the veggies start to turn golden, add a generous splash of water and simmer for a further three to five minutes, or until they are soft.

Step 4: In the remaining soy dressing, whisk in the cornflour and 1 tablespoon water. Transfer to a wok and let bubble for 30 seconds, stirring to coat everything in the sauce. Add the coriander, sesame seeds, and spring onion on top. Accompany with rice.

Chapter 5: Divine Desserts

1.DELICIOUS PISTACHIO MUFFINS WITHOUT PUDDING MIX

Prep time: 5 minutes
Cook time: 20 minutes
Serving: 12

Ingredients

Dry Flour Mixture
- 2 cups All-Purpose Flour
- 2 teaspoon Baking Powder • 1/2 teaspoon Salt
For the Wet Ingredients Mix
- 3/4 cup Granulated Sugar
- 1/2 cup Melted Unsalted Butter • 2 Large Eggs
- 3/4 cup Milk
- Lemon Zest of Half Lemon
- Food Coloring Optional
Additional Ingredients
- 1/4 cup Coarsley Powdered Pistachios • 1/4 cup Coarsley Powdered Mixed Nuts
For Decorating
- 3 oz Milk Chocolate
- 1/3 cup Chopped Pistachios • 1/3 cup Chopped Mixed Nuts

Directions

•The oven should be preheated to 400°F, 180°C fan, 200°C static or Gas Mark 6.

•Mix together the baking powder, salt, and sifted all-purpose flour in a bowl with the dry ingredients.

•All the wet ingredients should be combined in a bigger, separate bowl. These include the melted unsalted butter, eggs, sugar, milk, lemon zest, and food colouring, if needed.

•Three or four tablespoons of the dry ingredients should be added to the wet ones at a time, with mixing in between. Once everything is thoroughly combined, stop mixing (overmixing could make the muffins too dense).

•Place the mixed nuts and pistachios in the food processor and pulse until a coarse powder is achieved.

•Without overmixing, add the nut mixture to the muffin batter and stir until thoroughly combined.

•After filling each paper liner 2⁄3 to 3⁄4 full, add the muffin batter to the liners in the muffin tray.

•Oven bake the muffins for around 18 minutes (this will vary depending on the oven) on the centre shelf.

•When a toothpick is inserted or a cake tester is used, the muffins are done.

•When they're cooked, take the pistachio muffin pan out of the oven and allow it to cool for ten minutes on a wire rack.

•Ten minutes later, take the cupcakes out of the pan and let them cool fully on the rack. This will prevent the cupcake liners from becoming greasy due to moisture collecting at the bottom of them.

•In order to garnish the pistachio muffins, coarsely chop the leftover pistachios and mixed nuts. Meanwhile, melt the milk chocolate in a different mixing dish using a bain-marie or a microwave.

•When the chocolate is finished, dip the muffin domes into it before dipping them into the chopped pistachios and mixed nuts before it sets.

•Your muffins with green pistachios are prepared for serving.

2.EASY GOOEY BROWNIES

Prep time: 20 minutes
Cook time: 30 minutes
Serving: 20

Ingredients

- 150g butter
- 75g light soft brown sugar
- 150g plain chocolate, broken into pieces
- 1 tbsp golden syrup
- 3eggs
- 125g golden caster sugar
- 1 tsp vanilla extract
- 150g plain flour
- 1/2 tsp baking powder
- 3 tbsp cocoa powder, plus more to dust
- 4-6 tbsp dulce de leche, caramel or chocolate hazelnut spread

Directions

Step 1: Preheat the oven to 180°C (160°C for fans) or gas 4. Line a 20cm by 20cm cake tin with parchment paper. Gently melt the butter, chocolate, brown sugar, and golden syrup over low heat until a creamy consistency is achieved. Remove the pan from the hob.

Step 2: In a large bowl, whisk together the eggs and caster sugar until light and fluffy. It's important to do this well, as it will take a few minutes. Add the vanilla essence, then stir in the chocolate mixture after sifting in the flour, baking powder, and cocoa powder. Scatter half of the mixture into the tin and fold in the remaining ingredients rapidly. Spoon caramel or chocolate hazelnut spread onto the surface, then cover with the remaining brownie mixture.If desired, add more scoops of caramel or chocolate spread, then bake for 30 minutes. The mixture beneath will still wobble slightly, but the top of the mixture should now have set and seem somewhat cracked.

Step 3: Take out of the oven and let it cool fully before slicing it into squares. If you would like, dust the tops with cocoa powder or icing sugar. If you are serving them as dessert, drizzle with extra caramel. Will store in a sealed bag for up to three days.

3.STICKY TOFFEE PEAR PUDDING

Prep time: 25 minutes
Cook time: 50 minutes
Serving: 8

Ingredients

- 8 small firm pears (we used Conference)
- 200g golden caster sugar
- 2 cinnamon sticks
- 1 star anise
- 6 cloves
- 1 lemon, zest pared
- 1 orange, zest pared
- vegan ice cream, to serve (optional)

For the sponge

- 250g pitted dates
- 2 tbsp linseeds
- 300ml unsweetened almond milk
- 200ml vegetable oil, plus extra for greasing
- 175g dark muscovado sugar
- 200g self-raising flour
- 1 tsp bicarbonate of soda
- 1 tsp ground mixed spice

Directions

STEP 1: To create a level base, peel the pears and chop off the bottoms. Trim them to a height that allows your tin to fit inside tightly. Cut the pip pieces off of the base with a tiny knife. Chop the pear scraps coarsely, removing the pits, and reserve. Fill a pot big enough to hold all the pears with the sugar, cinnamon, star anise, cloves, zests, and 600ml of water. After bringing to a boil, simmer for the sugar to dissolve. When a knife easily inserts into a pear, add the pears, cover with a lid or a piece of baking parchment, and poach gently for 15 minutes. Allow the drink to chill you down.

STEP 2: Prepare the sponge now. Place the linseeds and dates in a saucepan, then pour in the almond milk. After bringing to a low boil, cook for two to three minutes, or until the dates are tender. Fill a food processor with the mixture and pulse until smooth. Blend in the oil once more, then scrape into a bowl and allow to cool somewhat. Preheat oven to 180°C (fan 160°C) and gas 4. Grease and line a 20 x 30 cm baking pan with a strip of baking parchment, preferably one with a loose bottom.

STEP 3: Combine the dry ingredients and 1/ 2 tsp salt in a large mixing bowl. Mix thoroughly, using your fingers to break up any sugar lumps, and shake the bowl a few times to help any lumps that remain rise to the surface. Stir thoroughly after adding the date and oil mixture. Add the chopped pear scraps and fold. Load the cake mixture into the tin, then carefully nestle the pears so that the bottom half are covered, standing straight up. Bake the cake for 35 to 40 minutes, or until it's done. To inspect, insert a skewer into the core; it should come out clean. Return the cake to the oven and bake it for ten minutes if the skewer shows any signs of moist cake mixture.

STEP 4: In the interim, return the liquid used to poach the pears to a boil and cook it until it reduces to a glossy syrup. Once the pudding is baked, allow it to cool for five to ten minutes before brushing it all over with the syrup. You can save some extra to serve with vegan ice cream if you'd like.

4.LEMON CHEESECAKE

Prep time: 20 minutes
 Cook time: 5 minutes
Serving: 6

Ingredients

- 110g digestive biscuits
- 50g butter
- 25g light brown soft sugar
- 350g mascarpone
- 75g caster sugar
- 1 lemon, zested
- 2-3 lemons, juiced (about 90ml)

Directions

Step 1: Use a rolling pin or a food processor to crush the digestive biscuits in a food bag. In a saucepan, melt the butter, remove from the heat, and mix in the biscuit crumbs and brown sugar.

Step 2: Use baking parchment to line the bottom of a 20cm loose-bottomed cake tin. While preparing the topping, press the biscuit firmly into the bottom of the tin and store it in the refrigerator.

 Step 3: Blend the mascarpone, caster sugar, zest, and juice of the lemon until it becomes smooth and creamy. Cover the base with it, then refrigerate for a few hours.

5.SUMMER PUDDING

Prep time: 20 minutes
Cook time: 10 minutes
Serving: 8

Ingredients

- 300g strawberry
- 250g blackberry
- 100g redcurrant
- 500g raspberry
- OR 1.25kg/2lb 12oz mixed berries and currants of your choice
- 175g golden caster sugar
- 7 slices day-old white bread, from a square, medium-cut loaf

Directions

Step 1: Extract juice: Clean the fruit and pat dry with a kitchen towel, making sure to keep the strawberries apart. In a big pan, combine sugar and 3 tablespoons water. Stirring occasionally, gently heat until sugar melts. After one minute of boiling, add the fruit (not strawberries). Cook over low heat for 3 minutes, stirring every 2 to 3 minutes. There will be a dark red fluid surrounding the softened, mostly intact fruit. Place a bowl over a sieve and pour the fruit and juice through it.

Step 2: Prepare the bread and cover the bowl with clingfilm: Cling film should be placed inside the 1.25-liter basin to facilitate turning out the pudding. It is simpler to overlap two pieces of cling film in the centre of the bowl than to attempt to get one sheet to adhere to every curve. Allow a 15cm overlap along the edges. Slice the bread in half. Cut four bread slices in half, slightly skewed so that each slice has two uneven rectangles. Slice 2 of the slices into 4 triangles each, leaving the remaining portion whole.

Step 3: Assemble the pudding: briefly submerge the entire bread slice in the juice to coat it. Press this into the basin's bottom. Dip each of the uneven rectangular pieces in the water, then press them around the edges of the basin until they fit together neatly, alternating between putting the wide and narrow ends up. It doesn't matter if the final piece of bread doesn't fit perfectly; just cut it into a triangle, dip it in juice, and slide it in. Spoon in the softened fruit now, sprinkling in the strawberries as you go.

Step 4: Allow tastes to meld before serving: After dipping the bread triangles in juice, stack them on top and use scissors to snip off the excess. Save any extra juice for later. Lift up the cling film and close it loosely. Place a side plate on top and use cans as weight. For six hours or overnight, chill. To serve, unfold the clingfilm, place a serving plate on top, then turn it over. Serve with cream, any remaining berries, and any leftover juice.

6.ROSEWATER AND RASPBERRY SPONGE CAKE

Prep time:35 minutes
Cook time:25 minutes
Serving:10-12

Ingredients

- 225g unsalted butter, softened, plus extra for greasing
- 225g golden caster sugar
- 4 medium eggs, beaten
- 1 tsp vanilla extract
- 225g self-raising flour, sifted For the rose cream filling
- 150ml double cream
- 1 tsp rosewater
- 4 tbsp raspberry jam
- 150g raspberries, slightly crushed

For the rose icing

- 175g icing sugar, plus extra for dusting
- 1/2 tsp rosewater

To decorate

- dried rose petals

Directions

STEP 1: Preheat oven to 180°C (160°C for fans or gas). 4. Grease two 20cm cake tins very lightly, then line them with baking parchment. In a large mixing basin, beat together the butter and sugar until light and fluffy. Add the eggs gradually, a bit at a time, scraping down the side of the bowl as you go. To prevent curdling, add 1 tsp flour to the mixture. Mix in half of the flour, fold in the remaining flour, and add the vanilla extract.

STEP 2: Split the batter among the cake pans and bake for twenty to twenty-five minutes; a skewer inserted in the centre of the cakes should come out clean.

STEP 3: Prepare the filler in the interim. Gently whisk the cream until it forms soft peaks, gradually incorporating the rosewater. Gently fold in the jam, taking care not to overmix.

STEP 4: Arrange a serving plate with a sponge on it, then cover it with the cream mixture. After scattering the raspberries, cover with the remaining sponge.

STEP 5: To make the icing, combine the icing sugar, rosewater, and two tablespoons of water. Then, add the juice of a few crushed raspberries. Drizzle over the cake, then arrange the leftover raspberries and rose petals.

7.ORANGE AND RHUBARB AMARETTI POTS

Prep time:10 minutes
Cook time:30 minutes
Serving:8

Ingredients

- 400g double cream
- 360g thick full-fat Greek yogurt
- 150g amaretti biscuits, broken into small pieces
For the rhubarb & orange curd
- 500g rhubarb, chopped into 2.5cm lengths
- 150g golden caster sugar, plus a large pinch
- 150ml orange juice, plus zest 1 orange
- 4 medium eggs, plus 2 medium yolks
- 150g unsalted butter

Directions

STEP 1: Make the curd first. Place the orange juice, rhubarb, and a little amount of sugar in a skillet over medium heat and cover. Cook until the rhubarb is very soft, about 10 to 15 minutes. Take off the heat source.

STEP 2: Push as much pulp out of the rhubarb as you can by passing it through a fine sieve. Save the meat in the strainer for subsequent incorporation.

STEP 3: Until pale and foamy, whisk together the eggs, egg yolks, and sugar. Gradually melt the butter in a pan over low heat. After melting, gradually whisk in the egg mixture and orange zest while swirling constantly. Stir in the strained rhubarb pulp and heat, stirring, until the curd thickens into a custard-like consistency. It can take ten to twelve minutes, so be patient and don't increase the heat lest you scramble the eggs.

STEP 4: Transfer the thickened curd to a bowl and whisk to make sure it's smooth. In order to give the dish more substance at this point, I like to put the rhubarb flesh back from the sieve; but, if you like a smooth curd,

STEP 5: Whip the cream until soft peaks form, pausing slightly before that happens. Stir in 300g of curd, the yoghurt, and the majority of the Ameretti biscuits.

STEP 6: Divide the mixture among eight glasses, then top with the saved amaretti. Keep the leftover curd for small tartlets, granola, or pancakes. Sterilise a jar by washing it in hot, soapy water, rinsing it and then baking it upside down at 120°C/100°F fan/gas 1/2 for 15 minutes to dry

8.BLUEBERRY AND COCONUT CAKE

Prep time:20 minutes
Cook time: 1hour 15 minutes
Serving:12

Ingredients

- 250ml rice bran oil, plus extra for the tin
- 3eggs
- 225g caster sugar
- 2 tsp vanilla extract
- 300g self-raising flour
- 50g desiccated coconut
- 175ml soya milk
- 140g fresh or frozen blueberries, plus extra to serve
- icing sugar, to dust

Directions

Step 1: Grease a 22cm Bundt or ring tin and preheat the oven to 180C/160C fan/gas 4. Whisk together the oil, eggs, sugar, and vanilla in a sizeable bowl. Mix the coconut and flour together. Alternatively, fold the flour mixture, beginning and ending with the flour, into the wet components together with the soy milk.

Step 2: Put a quarter into the canister. Spoon the remaining batter into the tin, then fold in the blueberries. A skewer put into the centre should come out clean after one and a half hours of baking. If the cake browns too rapidly, cover it with foil.

Step 3: Let cool in the tin for ten minutes, then transfer to a wire rack to finish cooling. To serve, place additional blueberries in the centre of the cake and sprinkle with powdered sugar.

Chapter 6: Satisfying Sides

1.SPICED ROAST SIDE OF SALMON

Prep time:10 minutes

Cook time:20 minutes

Serving:6

Ingredients

- 11/2 kg side of salmon, skin on
- 1 tbsp olive oil, plus extra for brushing
- 1/2 tsp ground ginger
- 1 tsp paprika
- 1/2 tsp coarsely ground black peppercorns
- 1 tbsp wholegrain mustard
- 1 tsp honey
- 1 lemon, cut into wedges, to serve

Directions

Step 1: Preheat oven to 200°C (180°C for fans or gas). 6. Use foil or baking paper to line a large roasting pan; this will assist keep the fish from sticking to the pan while it cooks. Place the salmon skin-side down on the paper after giving it a quick oil brushing.

Step 2: Combine the ground ginger with 1 tablespoon olive oil, paprika, pepper, mustard, and honey. Evenly distribute it on the fish's meaty side.

Step 3: Roast the salmon, uncovered, for about 20 minutes, or until it is cooked through. To check whether the salmon is done, pierce it with a knife and make sure it flake easily.

Step 4: Serve straight out of the tin, or delicately remove the salmon onto a large platter using a few fish slices.

2.CHICKPEA CURRY

Prep time:15 minutes
Cook time:25 minutes

Ingredients

- 2 tbsp oil
- 1 onion, diced
- 1 tsp fresh or dried chilli, to taste
- 9 garlic cloves (approx 1 small bulb of garlic)
- thumb-sized piece ginger, peeled
- 1 tbsp ground coriander
- 2 tbsp ground cumin
- 1 tbsp garam masala
- 2 tbsp tomato purée

For the curry

- 2 x 400g cans chickpeas, drained
- 400g can chopped tomatoes
- 100g creamed coconut
- 1⁄2 small pack coriander, chopped, plus extra to garnish
- 100g spinach

Directions

STEP 1: First, prepare the paste by heating a small amount of the 2 tablespoons oil in a frying pan, adding 1 diced onion and 1 tsp fresh or dried chilli, and cooking for about 8 minutes, or until softened.

STEP 2: Place 9 garlic cloves, a thumb-sized piece of peeled ginger, and the remaining oil in a food processor. Next, add 1 tablespoon each of ground coriander and cumin, 1 tablespoon of garam masala, 2 tablespoons of tomato purée, 1⁄2 teaspoon of salt, and the fried onion. Blend until a smooth consistency is achieved; add extra oil or a drop of water if necessary.

STEP 3: Cook the paste for two minutes over medium-high heat in a medium saucepan, stirring periodically to prevent sticking.

STEP 4: Add a 400g can of chopped tomatoes and two 400g cans of drained chickpeas. Simmer for five minutes to reduce the quantity.

STEP 5: Add 100g creamed coconut and a small pack of chopped coriander. Cook until the spinach wilts, about 5 more minutes.

STEP 6: Add more coriander as a garnish and serve with dhal or rice, preferably both.

3.VEGETARIAN GRAVY

Prep time:10 minutes
Cook time:35 minutes
Serving:6-8

Ingredients

- 1 onion, chopped
- 2 carrots, finely diced
- 2 celery sticks, finely chopped
- 2 bay leaves
- 1 large thyme sprig
- large knob of butter
- 1 tbsp sugar
- 2 tbsp plain flour
- 1 tsp Marmite (optional, but it does add colour and depth)
- 1 tbsp tomato purée
- 2 tbsp red wine vinegar
- 1l vegetable stock (or chicken or beef stock, if you prefer)

Directions

STEP 1: Fry the herbs and veggies in butter for ten to twelve minutes, or until the vegetables begin to brown. After adding the sugar, simmer until it becomes caramelised and sticky.

STEP 2: Add the tomato purée, vinegar, and Marmite, if using, and stir until the flour is sandy. After adding the stock, cover and boil everything until the sauce thickens.

STEP 3: Sieve, then season and colour with soy sauce. Use immediately, or let cool and freeze.

4.NAAN BREAD

Prep time:20 minutes
Cook time:35 minutes
Serving:7

Ingredients

- 1x 7g sachet dried yeast
- 2 tsp golden caster sugar
- 300g strong white bread flour, plus extra for dusting
- 1/2 tsp baking powder
- 25g butter or ghee, melted, plus extra 2-3 tbsp for the tray and brushing
- 150ml natural yogurt
- 1 tbsp nigella seeds

Directions

Step 1: Pour 125 millilitres of warm water into a bowl, then add 1 tsp of sugar and the yeast. Wait ten to fifteen minutes, or until foamy. Place the flour, remaining sugar, 1/2 teaspoon salt, and baking powder in a bigger bowl. Stir to combine, then create a well in the middle to add the yoghurt, melted butter, nigella seeds, and yeast mixture. After giving it a good stir, begin to incorporate the mixture with your hands. Add a teaspoon of flour if it's very moist, and a dash extra warm water if it's dry. The dough should be extremely soft, but not so moist that it cannot be formed into a ball.

Step 2: Once the consistency is satisfactory, begin kneading the mixture in the bowl and then move it to a surface that has been well-floured. Knead for ten minutes, or until the mixture is smooth and elastic but still soft. After buttering a big bowl, roll the dough into a ball and drop it into the bowl. Once it has doubled in size, cover and set in a warm location for around one hour.

Step 3: Form the dough into six balls, place them on a baking dish covered with a moist tea towel and sprinkled with flour. Over high heat, preheat a large nonstick frying pan. Roll out one of the dough balls to create a teardrop shape that is about 21 cm long and 13 cm broad at its widest point. The naan bread should be carefully placed into the heated pan. Allow it to dry fry and puff up for about 3 minutes. Then, turn it over and cook for an additional 3–4 minutes on the other side, or until it's cooked through and has some char on it.

Step 4: Place the cooked naan bread on a baking pan and preheat the oven to the lowest temperature possible. Apply a thin layer of melted butter and securely wrap with foil. As you prepare the naans, keep them warm in the oven and stack them on top of one another, coating each one with melted butter or ghee. Warm up and serve with dips or curries.

5.CHAPATIS

Prep time:15 minutes
Cook time:10 minutes
Serving:10

Ingredients

- 140g wholemeal flour
- 140g plain flour, plus extra for dusting
- 1 tsp salt
- 2 tbsp olive oil, plus extra for greasing
- 180ml hot water or as needed

Directions

Step 1: Combine the flours and salt in a big bowl. Add enough water and olive oil with a wooden spoon to form a soft, elastic, but not sticky dough.

Step 2: Until the dough is smooth, knead it for five to ten minutes on a surface dusted with flour. Cut into ten equal pieces, or fewer if you prefer larger loaves. Shape each component into a ball. Take a few minutes to rest.

Step 3: Lightly grease and heat a frying pan over medium heat. Roll out the dough balls with a floured rolling pin on a lightly floured board until they are very thin, like a tortilla.

Step 4: Place a chapati on the pan once it begins to smoke. Cook for about 30 seconds, or until there are brown spots on the underside, then turn and cook the other side. Transfer to a plate and keep warm while preparing the remaining chapatis.

6.SPICY PANEER SKEWERS

Prep time:15 minutes
Cook time:10 minutes
Serving:10

Ingredients

- 600g paneer cheese (see Tip below)
- juice 2 lemons
- 2 tsp ground cumin, plus extra for sprinkling
- 75g gram flour (see Tip below)
- 1 tsp garam masala
- 1 tbsp paprika
- 284ml tub double cream
- 4 garlic cloves, crushed
- 2 red chillies, deseeded and chopped
- 2 peppers, red and yellow, roughly chopped
- 2 courgettes, sliced
- 25g butter, melted
- 2 lemons, cut into wedges

Directions

Step 1: To prevent the bamboo skewers from burning beneath the grill, soak them in water for 15 minutes. Chop the paneer cheese into cubes about 3 cm, then mix it with the ground cumin and lemon juice. Put away for half an hour.

Step 2: Transfer the gramme flour, paprika, and garam masala to a bowl. Add the cream, chopped chilies, garlic, and enough water to create a thick batter. Stir until smooth. After draining the paneer,
combine it with two tablespoons of the lemon juice infused with cumin. Apply batter to each and every paneer cube.

Step 3: Close the grill lid and preheat the grill to its highest temperature. Place the paneer and chunks of pepper and courgette

alternately onto skewers. Pour in batter from the bowl, then cook for 4–5 minutes on each side, turning them over and spooning in additional batter. Grill until the edges get blackened. Serve right away with lemon slices, brush with melted butter, and sprinkle with ground cumin.

7.BANANA BREAD

Prep time:15 minutes
Cook time:50 minutes
Serving:8-10 slices

Ingredients

- 140g butter, softened, plus extra for the tin
- 140g caster sugar
- 2 large eggs, beaten
- 140g self-raising flour
- 1 tsp baking powder
- 2 very ripe bananas, mashed
- 50g icing sugar
- handful dried banana chips, for decoration

Directions

Step 1: Preheat oven to 180°C (160°C for fans or gas). 4.

Step 2: Grease a 2-pound loaf pan and place baking paper inside the pan's bottom and edges.

Step 3: Beat 2 big eggs with a bit of the 140g flour and gently add to the 140g melted butter and 140g caster sugar until light and fluffy.

Step 4: Stir in 2 mashed bananas, 1 tsp baking powder, and the remaining flour.

Step 5: Transfer the mixture into the prepared pan and bake for approximately fifty minutes, or until thoroughly done. The loaf may take a different amount of time depending on the form of your loaf pan, so check it every 5 minutes for 30 to 40 minutes by sticking a skewer in and ensuring that it emerges clean.

Step 6: After 10 minutes of cooling in the tin, remove to a wire rack.

Step 7: To prepare a runny frosting, combine 50g of icing sugar with 2-3 tsp water.

Step 8: Spread the frosting over the cake's top and garnish with a few banana chips.

8.PINEAPPLE FRIED RICE

Prep time:10 minutes
Cook time:10 minutes
Serving:4

Ingredients

- 11/2 tbsp sunflower or vegetable oil
- 2 eggs, beaten
- 2 garlic cloves, crushed
- small bunch of spring onions, chopped
- 1/2 tsp Chinese five-spice powder
- 400g cooked long-grain rice
- 85g frozen peas
- 2 tsp sesame oil
- 2 tbsp low-salt soy sauce
- 400g fresh pineapple, roughly chopped into chunks (about 1/2 medium pineapple)

Directions

Step 1: In a wok, heat up one tablespoon of oil. In order to create a thin omelette, add the eggs and swirl them up the sides. After the omelette is fully cooked, roll it out onto a cutting board and cut it into ribbons.

Step 2: Warm up the leftover oil. Add the onions, garlic, and five spice. Add the rice (if using pouches, squeeze them first to separate the grains), peas, sesame oil, and soy and stir-fry until sizzling. Cook on high heat until the rice is heated through, then mix in the omelette ribbons and pineapple.

9.VEGGIE KOFTA PITTAS WITH PICK AND MIX SIDES

Prep time:20 minutes
Cook time:30 minutes
Serving:6

Ingredients

- 2 onions, chopped
- 2 garlic cloves, crushed
- 1 Cal cooking spray, for frying
- 2 x 400g cans chickpeas, drained
- 100g fresh brown breadcrumbs
- 1 large egg
- 2 tsp ground cumin
- 2 tsp ground coriander
- zest 1 lemon, 1 tbsp juice, plus extra wedges to serve
- 85g baby spinach
- toasted pitta breads, to serve
- 175g fat-free natural or Greek yogurt, to serve
- pickled chillies or jalapeños (optional), to serve

For the carrot & tomato salad
- 200g carrots, coarsely grated
- 200g tomatoes, diced
- 1/2 red onion, finely chopped
- 2 tbsp red wine vinegar
- 1 tsp sugar

Directions

STEP 1: In a nonstick pan, soften the garlic and onions with a couple sprays of 1 Cal cooking spray and a drop of water. Once very soft, transfer to a food processor along with the breadcrumbs, egg, spices, zest and juice of lemon, and enough of seasoning for the chickpeas. Add 30g of the spinach and pulse until finely chopped after pulsing until reasonably smooth. Form the mixture into 12 sausage-shaped koftas and place on a baking tray fitted with parchment paper. As you preheat the oven to 200°C (180°F for fans) or gas 6.

STEP 2: Continue to coat the koftas with cooking spray a few times, and bake for 20 to 25 minutes, or until they are crisp and golden.

STEP 3 Combine all the ingredients for the carrot salad and season to taste. Transfer the leftover spinach to a bowl and reheat the pittas as directed on the package.

STEP 4: If desired, serve the koftas with warm pita bread, extra spinach, carrot salad, fat-free yoghurt, and pickled chilies.

Chapter 7: Hearty Soups and Stews

1. BUTTERNUT SQUASH CHIPOTLE CHILLI WITH AVOCADO

Prep time:20 minutes
Cook time: 1hour
Serving:4

Ingredients

- 2 tablespoons olive oil
- 1 medium red onion, chopped
- 2 red bell peppers, chopped
- 1 small butternut squash (1 1⁄2 pounds or less), peeled and chopped into 1⁄2-inch cubes
- 4 garlic cloves, pressed or minced
- 1 tablespoon chili powder
- 1⁄2+ tablespoon chopped chipotle pepper in adobo* (start with 1⁄2 tablespoon and add more to taste, I thought mine was just right with 1 tablespoon)
- 1 teaspoon ground cumin
- 1⁄4 teaspoon ground cinnamon
- 1 bay leaf
- 2 cans (15 ounces each) black beans, rinsed and drained, or 3 cups cooked black beans
- 1 small can (14 ounces) diced tomatoes, including the liquid**
- 2 cups vegetable broth (or one 14-ounce can)
- Salt, to taste
- 2 Avocados from Mexico, diced
- 3 corn tortillas for crispy tortilla strips (or substitute crumbled tortilla chips)
- Optional additional garnishes: Chopped fresh cilantro and/or red pepper flakes

Directions

•Heat the olive oil in a 4- to 6-quart Dutch oven or stockpot over medium heat until it shimmers. Stirring occasionally, add the onion, bell pepper, and butternut squash and simmer until the onions become translucent.

•Reduce the heat to medium-low and mix in the cinnamon, cumin, 1/2 tablespoon chopped chipotle peppers, chilli powder, and garlic. Cook for about 30 seconds, stirring regularly, or until aromatic. Add the broth, tomatoes with their juices, black beans, and bay leaf. After combining, cover and stir occasionally for approximately one hour. About halfway through cooking, taste and adjust seasoning with more chopped chipotle peppers, if desired.

•When the butternut squash is perfectly soft and the liquid has somewhat reduced to create that classic, hearty chilli consistency, you'll know your chilli is ready. After removing the bay leaf, season with salt.

•To prepare the crunchy tortilla strips, stack the corn tortillas and cut them into thin, 1/4-inch-wide by 2-inch-long strips. In a medium pan, warm a drizzle of olive oil over medium heat until it shimmers. Add the tortilla slices, mix, and sprinkle with salt. Cook, stirring periodically, until the strips are crispy and turning brown, 4 to 7 minutes. Take out the tortilla strips from the skillet and place them on a paper towel-covered plate to drain.

•Present the chilli in separate bowls, garnished with a generous amount of cubed avocado and crunchy tortilla strips. I optionally added a tiny pinch of red pepper flakes. It would also be excellent with cilantro. For those of us who are addicted to spices like myself, you might want to serve this with some chipotle spicy sauce (Tobasco produces one).

2.CLASSIC MINESTRONE SOUP

Prep time:20 minutes
Cook time:45 minutes
Serving:6

Ingredients

- 4 tablespoons extra-virgin olive oil, divided
- 1 medium yellow onion, chopped
- 2 medium carrots, peeled and chopped
- 2 medium ribs celery, chopped
- 1/4 cup tomato paste
- 2 cups chopped seasonal vegetables (potatoes, yellow squash, zucchini, butternut squash, green beans or peas all work)
- 4 cloves garlic, pressed or minced
- 1/2 teaspoon dried oregano
- 1/2 teaspoon dried thyme
- 1 large can (28 ounces) diced tomatoes, with their liquid (or 2 small 15-ounce cans)
- 4 cups (32 ounces) vegetable broth
- 2 cups water
- 1 teaspoon fine sea salt
- 2 bay leaves
- Pinch of red pepper flakes
- Freshly ground black pepper
- 1 cup whole grain orecchiette, elbow or small shell pasta
- 1 can (15 ounces) Great Northern beans or cannellini beans, rinsed and drained, or 1 1/2 cups cooked beans
- 2 cups baby spinach, chopped kale or chopped collard greens
- 2 teaspoons lemon juice
- Freshly grated Parmesan cheese, for garnishing (optional)

Directions

•In a big stockpot or Dutch oven, preheat 3 tablespoons of olive oil over medium heat. Add the chopped onion, carrot, celery, tomato paste, and a dash of salt once the oil is shimmering. Cook for 7 to 10 minutes, stirring frequently, or until the veggies are tender and the onions are starting to become translucent.

•Add the thyme, oregano, garlic, and seasonal veggies. Cook for about 2 minutes, stirring regularly, or until aromatic.

•Add the water, broth, and diced tomatoes with their juices. Add the red pepper flakes, bay leaves, and salt. Add a lot of freshly ground black pepper for seasoning.

•Increase the heat to medium-high, bring the mixture to a boil, and then place a lid on the pot, leaving about an inch open to allow steam to escape. As needed, turn down the heat to keep a low simmer.

•After cooking for fifteen minutes, take off the lid and mix in the pasta, greens, and beans. Simmer, uncovered, for another 20 minutes or until the greens are soft and the pasta is cooked al dente.

•After taking the saucepan off of the hob, discard the bay leaves. Add the remaining tablespoon of olive oil and the lemon juice and stir. Once the flavours truly come together, taste and add more salt and pepper (I generally put about 1/4 tsp more). If desired, sprinkle grated Parmesan cheese over soup dishes.

3.WEST AFRICAN PEANUT SOUP

Prep time:10 minutes
Cook time:35 minutes
Serving:4

Ingredients

- 4 cups low-sodium vegetable broth
- 2 cups water
- 1 medium red onion, chopped
- 2 tablespoons peeled and minced fresh ginger
- 4 cloves garlic, minced
- 1 teaspoon salt
- 1 bunch collard greens (or kale), ribs removed and leaves chopped
into 1-inch strips
- 3⁄4 cup unsalted peanut butter (chunky or smooth)
- 1⁄2 cup tomato paste*
- Hot sauce, like sriracha (AKA rooster sauce)
- 1⁄4 cup roughly chopped peanuts, for garnish
- Cooked brown rice, for serving (optional)

Directions

•In a stock pot or medium Dutch oven, combine the broth and water. After bringing the mixture to a boil, whisk in the salt, garlic, ginger, and onion. Cook on medium-low heat for twenty minutes.

•Place 1 to 2 cups of the boiling stock in a medium-sized, heat-safe mixing bowl, and mix in the tomato paste and peanut butter. After smoothing out the mixture with a whisk, return the peanut mixture to the soup and thoroughly stir. Add the collard greens and taste and add more spicy sauce to the broth.

•Simmer over medium-low heat for approximately 15 more minutes, stirring frequently. If preferred, add more salt or spicy sauce for seasoning. If desired, place over cooked brown rice and garnish with a dusting of chopped peanuts.

4.CREAMY ROASTED CARROT SOUP

Prep time:15 minutes

Cook time:50 minutes

Serving:4

Ingredients

- 2 pounds carrots
- 3 tablespoons extra-virgin olive oil, divided
- 3⁄4 teaspoon fine sea salt, divided, to taste
- 1 medium yellow onion, chopped
- 2 cloves garlic, pressed or minced
- 1⁄2 teaspoon ground coriander
- 1⁄4 teaspoon ground cumin
- 4 cups vegetable broth (or water)
- 2 cups water
- 1 to 2 tablespoons unsalted butter, to taste
- 1 1⁄2 teaspoons lemon juice, to taste
- Freshly ground black pepper, to taste

Directions

•Set the oven's temperature to 400 degrees. If wanted, easily clean a big rimmed baking sheet by lining it with parchment paper.

•Peel and chop your carrots on the diagonal so that the broadest section of each slice is about 1⁄2″ thick (see photographs).

•Carrots should be put on the baking sheet. Add half a teaspoon of salt and two tablespoons of olive oil. Add oil and salt and toss until the carrots are lightly coated. Put them in an individual layer.

•Roast the carrots for 25 to 40 minutes, flipping them halfway through, or until the edges are caramelised and a fork can easily pierce them. (Heirloom carrot varieties can roast in 25 minutes, but normal carrots need 35 to 40 minutes to roast since they are denser.)

•When the carrots are almost done roasting, heat the remaining 1 tablespoon of olive oil in a Dutch oven or soup pot over medium heat until it shimmers. Combine the onion with a tsp of salt. Cook for 5 to 7 minutes, stirring occasionally, or until the onion is cooked and starting to turn translucent.

•Add the cumin, coriander, and garlic (see to the recipe notes if you're following a variant). Cook for 30 to 1 minute, stirring regularly, or until aromatic. Using a wooden spoon or robust silicone spatula, scrape out any browned bits from the bottom of the pan before adding the vegetable broth and water.
•After taking them out of the oven, add the roasted carrots to the soup. Over high fire, bring the mixture to a boil, then lower the heat.Cook for 15 minutes, to give the flavors time to meld.

•After the soup is cooked, take the pot off of the hob and allow it to cool for a short while. The heated soup should then be gently transferred—you may need to work in batches—to a blender. (The soup may overflow if you fill it past the maximum fill line.)

•Add the butter, squeeze in the lemon (or lime, if you're doing the Thai version), and grind in a few black peppercorns. Process till very smooth. If needed, taste and add more salt and pepper. If you want it to have more flavour, add a bit more lemon juice, or another tablespoon of butter. Blend one more before serving.

•This soup can be stored for several months in the freezer or for approximately four days in the refrigerator, covered.

5.FIVE-A-DAY TAGINE

Prep time:10 minutes
Cook time:35 minutes
Serving:4

Ingredients

- 4 carrots, cut into chunks
- 4 small parsnips, or 3 large, cut into chunks
- 3 red onions, cut into wedges
- 2 red peppers, deseeded and cut into chunks
- 2 tbsp olive oil
- 1 tsp each ground cumin, paprika, cinnamon and mild chilli powder
- 400g can chopped tomato
- 2 small handfuls soft dried apricots
- 2 tsp honey

Directions

STEP 1: Preheat the oven to 200°C (fan 180°C) or gas. 6. Divide the vegetables over two baking trays, sprinkle with half of the oil, season, and then use your hands to coat the vegetables with the oil. Roast until soft and starting to turn brown, about 30 minutes.

STEP 2: Fry the spices for a minute in the remaining oil; they should crackle and begin to smell wonderful. Add the can of water, honey, apricots, and tomatoes. Add the vegetables and spices after simmering for 5 minutes, or until the sauce has slightly reduced and the apricots have plumped up. Accompany with jacket potatoes or couscous.

6.TOMATO AND COURGETTE STEW

Prep time:10 minutes
Cook time: 1hour
Serving:4

Ingredients

- 1 tbsp olive oil
- 1 onion, chopped
- 2 garlic cloves, crushed
- 3 courgettes, quartered lengthways and cut into chunks
- 2 x 400g cans chopped tomatoes
- small bunch basil, torn
- 25g parmesan (or vegetarian alternative), finely grated

Directions

STEP 1: Place a big frying pan over medium heat and add oil. Add the onion and simmer until softened and beginning to turn golden brown, about 10 minutes. Cook for an additional five minutes after adding the garlic.

STEP 2: Add the courgettes and heat until they begin to soften, around 5 minutes. Add the tomatoes and thoroughly mix everything together. Add the basil and Parmesan after simmering for 35 to 40 minutes, or until the tomatoes have reduced and the courgettes are tender.

7.BEEF STEW

Prep time:15 minutes
Cook time:3 hours 50 minutes
Serving:5

Ingredients

- 2 celery sticks, thickly sliced
- 1 onion, chopped
- 2 really big carrots, halved lengthways then very chunkily sliced
- 5 bay leaves
- 2 thyme sprigs, 1 whole and 1 leaves picked
- 1 tbsp vegetable oil
- 1 tbsp butter
- 2 tbsp plain flour
- 2 tbsp tomato purée
- 2 tbsp Worcestershire sauce
- 2 beef stock cubes, crumbled
- 850g stewing beef (feather blade or brisket works nicely), cut into
nice large chunks

Directions

STEP 1: Turn on the kettle and preheat the oven to 160°C (140°F for fans) or gas 3.

STEP 2: Combine 1 tablespoon of butter and 1 tablespoon of vegetable oil in a flameproof casserole dish together with 2 thickly sliced celery sticks, 1 chopped onion, 2 chunkily sliced carrots, 5 bay leaves, and 1 full thyme sprig.

 STEP 3: After letting it soften for ten minutes, mix in two tablespoons plain flour until it stops looking dusty. Then, add two tablespoons tomato purée, two tablespoons Worcestershire sauce, and two crumbled beef stock cubes.

STEP 4: Stir in 600ml of boiling water gradually, then add 850g of stewing meat and cook gently.

STEP 5: After the meat is very soft and the sauce has thickened, cover and bake for 2 hours and 30 minutes. Then, uncover and continue cooking for an additional 30 to 1 hour.

STEP 6: Add the chopped leaves from the remaining thyme sprig as a garnish.

8.PUMPKIN STEW
Prep time:25 minutes
Cook time:2hours 20 minutes
 Serving:6

Ingredients

- 2 tbsp vegetable oil
- 500g stewing beef, cut into chunks
- 2 onions, sliced or chopped
- 600g carrots, cut into chunks
- 1 celery stick, roughly sliced
- 1/4 small bunch of thyme
- 2 bay leaves
- 1 1/2 tbsp tomato purée
- 1 1/2 tbsp plain flour
- 1 l vegetable stock
- 250ml ale or beer
- 1 medium pumpkin (about 500g), peeled, deseeded and chopped
- mashed potato or crusty bread, to serve

Directions

STEP 1: In a large, covered pan or flameproof casserole, heat the oil and cook the meat, in batches, over medium-high heat for a few minutes, or until browned. Transfer to a bowl and place it there. In the same pan, fry the onion for 6 to 8 minutes, or until it becomes tender.

 STEP 2: Cook for a few more minutes to soften the carrots and celery, stirring in the bay, thyme, and carrots. Put the steak back in the pan and stir in the flour and tomato purée.

STEP 3: Add the ale and stock, season to taste, and then bring to a boil. Simmer the mixture for one hour on low heat. Once the beef and vegetables are cooked, stir in the pumpkin and simmer for 30 to 1 hour. Serve with crusty bread or mashed potatoes to sop up the gravy.

9.SMOKY CHICKEN,BEAN AND KALE STEW

Prep time:10 minutes
Cook time: 1hour 25 minutes
Serving:4

Ingredients

- 1 tbsp olive oil
- 8 boneless and skinless chicken thighs
- 80g cubed pancetta or smoky bacon lardons
- 1 large red onion
- 4 pancetta
- 2 tsp smoked paprika
- 2 bay leaves
- 1 tbsp red wine vinegar
- 2 x 400g can plum tomatoes
- 1 tsp caster sugar
- 1 chicken stock cube
- 400g can cannellini or butter beans, drained
- 100g kale, stripped from the stalk and roughly chopped
- garlic bread, to serve
- drizzle of extra virgin olive oil (optional)

Directions

STEP 1: Fill a large casserole pan with heated oil. To prevent the skillet from becoming too crowded, add the chicken and cook it for a few minutes on each side, or until it turns golden brown. After removing the chicken, set it aside.

STEP 2: Cook the pancetta for 5 minutes, or until it begins to crisp. After pushing to one side, add the onion and simmer for about 8 minutes, or until softened. After adding the garlic, cook for an additional minute.

 STEP 3: Combine the vinegar, sugar, paprika, bay, and tomatoes. Finally, crumble in the stock cube. Replace the chicken in the pan after adding two cans full of water (800 ml), seasoning, and tasting. For thirty minutes, simmer with a lid on over low heat; bubbles should only occasionally appear.

STEP 4: After the stew has reduced to a rich soup, uncover the pan and continue cooking for an additional 30 minutes. By now the tomatoes should have broken down, but use the back of a wooden spoon to smash them if they're still very chunky. To separate the larger pieces of chicken, use two forks.

STEP 5: Stir the beans and kale into the stew, place a lid on it, and cook for five minutes to fully heat the beans and wilt the greens. If desired, top each serving of garlic bread chunks and deep bowls with a drizzle of high-quality extra virgin olive oil. Allow the stew to cool fully before transferring it to a freezer-safe container. keeps for a maximum of three months.

10.CREAMY CHICKEN STEW

Prep time:10 minutes
Cook time:55 minutes
Serving:4-6

Ingredients

- 3 leeks, halved and finely sliced
- 2 tbsp olive oil, plus extra if needed
- 1 tbsp butter
- 8 small chicken thighs
- 500ml chicken stock
- 1 tbsp Dijon mustard
- 75g crème fraîche
- 200g frozen peas
- 3 tbsp dried or fresh breadcrumbs
- small bunch of parsley, finely chopped

Directions

Step 1: Place the leeks, oil, and butter in a flameproof casserole dish over low heat. Cook, stirring constantly, for ten minutes, or until the leeks are tender.

Step 2: In a large nonstick frying pan, place the chicken skin-side down. Cook over medium heat until the skin turns brown, then flip it over and brown the other side. Although it shouldn't be necessary use a little oil if the skin begins to stick. Leaving any grease in the pan, add the chicken to the leeks.

Step 3: Pour in the stock, bring to a simmer, season well, cover, and cook on low for 30 minutes. Bring to a simmer after adding the peas, crème fraîche, and mustard. There should be a good amount of sauce on you.
Step 4: Light the grill when it's time to serve. Combine the breadcrumbs and parsley, then coat the chicken with them and cook it until it turns golden brown.

Chapter 8: Quick and Easy Meals

1.HERBY WARM CUCUMBERS WITH LEMON

Prep time:10 minutes
Cook time:4 minutes
 Serving:4

Ingredients

2 tbsp olive oil
small handful of mint, chopped
2 cucumbers, cut into thin ribbons using a vegetable peeler small handful of dill, chopped
small handful of parsley, chopped
1/2 lemon zested and juiced

Directions

STEP 1: Heat oil in a large saucepan. Cook the chopped mint for one minute. Then, add the cucumber ribbons and stir gently. Toss and cook for a further two to three minutes to reheat.

STEP 2: Turn off the heat and stir in the parsley, dill, and a splash of lemon juice. Transfer to a serving dish, top with additional lemon juice and lemon zest if desired.

2.KAJU KATLI

Prep time:30 minutes
Cook time:15 minutes
Serving:20

Ingredients

- 1 1/2 tbsp ghee, melted, a little extra for rolling
- 250g unsalted cashews
- 175g white sugar
- 1 pinch of saffron threads
- 1/4 tsp ground cardamom

Directions

- STEP 1:

Spread 1/2 tbsp of ghee on a shallow baking pan (ours measured 30cm by 20cm) after lining it with baking parchment. Put aside. Place the cashews in a skillet and toast them gently for three to four minutes, stirring them frequently to prevent browning and burning. After toasting, remove from the heat source and place onto a plate to cool.

- Step 2:

Place the cooled, roasted cashews in tiny batches into a powerful food processor and pulse just three times, or at very short intervals. It
is crucial to avoid grinding for an extended period of time, as this may cause the oil to escape and get lumpy and sticky. When the powder is light and fine, transfer it into a sieve placed over a bowl and gently sift. Until all of the cashews are ground fine enough to pass through the sieve, blitz the larger bits one more and filter according to the previous method.

- Step 3:

Heat a medium-sized frying pan to medium and add the sugar and
80ml water. Gently simmer, stirring when it begins to bubble. After the sugar has melted, which should take two to three minutes, turn down the heat and gradually whisk in the cashew powder using a spatula. Add the powder and stir thoroughly to remove any lumps. Add the ground cardamom and the saffron threads and stir. Stirring occasionally, cook for a further five minutes. Stir in 1 tablespoon of ghee after adding it. The mixture will start to thicken into the consistency of thick liquid fudge after 8 to 10 minutes.

● STEP 4:

To ensure the mixture is ready, take a tiny tablespoon of the dough, let it cool for five minutes, and then roll the cooled dough between your fingers while rubbing a ghee pinch made with your thumb and forefinger. It should not stick and roll readily into a ball. In the event that it does stick, cook the mixture for a few more minutes on low heat. Spread the dough out on the tray and cook for about 15 minutes, or until it's still warm but not too hot to handle.

● Step 5:

Apply a small amount of ghee to your palm, knead the dough for a minute (it should feel like soft fudge), and then slowly start to press it into a small circle with your fingers. Drizzle a small amount of ghee onto the pressed dough. Roll the dough out with a rolling pin until it is roughly the thickness of one centimetre.

● STEP 6:

Using a pizza cutter or sharp knife, cut through the square in 3 cm diagonals in both directions to form the flattened dough into diamond shapes. It is now ready to serve; the kaju katli just needs to sit at room temperature for about an hour. They ought to be set at a consistency similar to soft fudge.

3.GNOCCHI CACIO E PEPE

Prep time:2 minutes
Cook time:5 minutes
Serving:2

Ingredients

- 300g gnocchi
- 2 tbsp unsalted butter
- 60g parmesan or vegetarian alternative, finely grated
- 2 tsp black pepper
- salad leaves, to serve (optional)

Directions

STEP 1: Boil a big pan of water with a small amount of salt and cook the gnocchi. Retain 200ml of the cooking water by draining it.

STEP 2: In a sizable frying pan, melt the butter. Stir in 150ml of the cooking water, the gnocchi, cheese, and pepper. Increase the heat a little and stir quickly until the cheese melts and the gnocchi are thoroughly coated. If you prefer it saucier, add more of the saved water. Toss in a pinch of salt. Spoon the gnocchi into bowls and, if desired, accompany with a mixed salad.

4.PEA AND LEEK OPEN LASAGNE

Prep time:10 minutes
Cook time:15 minutes
 Serving:2

Ingredients

- 2 tbsp rapeseed oil
- 2 leeks, washed and sliced into half moons
- 2 garlic cloves, finely chopped
- 250g frozen peas
- 100g kale
- 1 tbsp wholegrain mustard
- 2 tbsp low-fat crème fraîche
- 1 lemon, zested
- 4 fresh lasagne sheets

Directions

Step1: Heat a frying pan to a medium temperature. Add a small teaspoon of salt, the garlic, and leeks to the oil. Cook, stirring now and then, until soft and collapsed. In the interim, heat up a pan of water.

Step 2: Add a splash of water and toss the kale and peas into the pan with the leeks. Simmer until the peas have defrosted and the kale has begun to wilt. Reduce the heat to a minimum. Add the crème fraîche,
 mustard, and half of the lemon zest and stir. Water should be added to create a sauce. Mix everything well and adjust the seasoning to taste.

Step 3: Lower the lasagna into the water and cook it as directed on the package; make sure to drain thoroughly. Arrange a single lasagna sheet onto each plate, followed with half of the leek and pea mixture, and then arrange the second lasagna sheet and the leftover greens on top. Sprinkle the leftover lemon zest over top and generously grind some black pepper.

5.INDIAN CHICKPEAS WITH POACHED EGGS

Prep time:5 minutes
Cook time:10 minutes
Serving:2

Ingredients

1 tbsp rapeseed oil
 2 garlic cloves, chopped
1 yellow pepper, deseeded and diced
1/2 - 1 red chilli, chopped and deseeded
1/2 bunch of spring onions (about 5), sliced, keeping the whites and tops apart 1 tsp cumin plus a little extra to serve (optional)
1 tsp coriander
1/2 tsp turmeric
3 tomatoes, cut into wedges
1/3 pack coriander, chopped
400g can of rinsed but reserved liquid chickpeas in water
1/2 teaspoon powdered reduced-salt bouillon (Marigold)
4 large eggs

Directions

Step 1: Heat the oil in a nonstick sauté pan, then add the spring onion whites, garlic, pepper, and chilli. Fry for five minutes over medium-high heat. In the meantime, bring a big pan of water to a boil.

Step 2: Fill the sauté pan with the spices, tomatoes, chickpeas, and most of the coriander. Simmer for a further 30 to 40 seconds. After adding enough liquid from the chickpeas to cover everything, stir in the bouillon powder and reduce the heat to low.

 Step 3: Crack in your eggs and poach for two minutes, then remove with a slotted spoon once the water is a rolling boil. After adding the spring onion tops to the chickpeas, gently mash a handful of them using a fork or potato masher. Transfer the chickpea mixture onto plates, garnish with the eggs, and sprinkle with the saved coriander. If desired, top the dish with an additional sprinkle of cumin.

Chapter 9: Refreshing Beverages

1.NON-DAIRY CINNAMON VANILLA CASHEW MILK

Prep time:5 minutes
Serving:4 cups

Ingredients

- 1 cup raw cashews soaked for at least 4 hours
- 3 cups water
- 2 tbsp Grade B maple syrup more if you want it sweeter • 1 tsp ground cinnamon
- 1 vanilla bean cut and scraped

Directions

• Mix all ingredients in a blender until smooth. If you have a powerful blender, it should be easy to get the cashew milk perfectly smooth; if not, just filter the milk through a fine mesh strainer or cheesecloth before serving.

2.RASPBERRY BANANA CHIA SMOOTHIE

Prep time: 5 minutes
Serving:1

Ingredients

- 1 cup vanilla or chocolate flavoured non-dairy milk
- 1 tbsp chia seeds
- 1/4 cup frozen raspberries
- 1 frozen banana half
- sweetener of choice to taste if desired

Directions

- In a blender, combine milk and chia seeds. Give it five minutes to sit.

- Blend in half of the banana and the raspberries until smooth. • If desired, add sweetener after tasting.

3.DALGONA WHIPPED COFFEE

Prep time: 5 minutes
Serving:1

Ingredients

- 2 tbsp boiling water
- 2 tbsp sugar
- 2 tbsp instant coffee
- 1 1/2 cups milk or your favourite plant-based milk for a
vegan version

Directions

- Fill a medium mixing bowl with the sugar, instant coffee, and hot water. Note: As you whisk, the mixture will seem to require a lot smaller bowl, but it really gets bigger.

- Whisk until the mixture thickens and takes on the consistency of yoghurt.

- Fill a cup almost to the brim with ice.

- Pour the milk into the cup until it's about three-quarters full.

- When the cup is about full, spoon the whipped coffee mixture on top. (Your finished drink will taste richer the more creamed coffee you add.)

- Using a straw, stir until nearly all of the whipped coffee and milk is mixed.

4.PINEAPPLE JALAPEÑO GRANITA

Prep time:20 minutes
Cook time:3 hours
Serving:8

Ingredients

- 1 cup water
- 1⁄2 cup white sugar (organic for vegan-friendly)
- 1 jalapeño halved (don't discard the seeds)
- 1 lb pineapple peeled and diced
- juice from 1 lime
- 1⁄2 tsp salt

Directions

- In a small saucepan, combine the water, sugar, and jalapeño; simmer over medium-high heat, stirring often. Reduce heat and simmer for an additional five minutes once the mixture reaches a boil.
- After allowing the mixture to reach room temperature, strain it through a fine-mesh sieve.
- Process the pineapple, sugar mixture, lime juice, and salt in a food processor until smooth.
- Fill 9 x 13-inch baking pan with ingredients. Freeze until the edges start to solidify with ice. Once again, invert and freeze for a further 20 to 30 minutes, stirring with a fork until the granita is fully frozen.
- Serve the granita by using a fork to shave it into fluffy crystals.

5.STRAWBERRY MANGO FIZZ SMOOTHIE

Prep time:5 minutes
Serving:1

Ingredients

- 1/2 cup mango sorbet
- 1/4 cup strawberries frozen or fresh both work
- 1/2 cup sparkling water I'm using citrus flavoured water in a blender.

Directions

- Process (with an immersion blender for easy cleanup) and then serve and savour!

6.FIVE-MINUTES DELICIOUS EGGNOG

Prep time:5 minutes
Serving:4

Ingredients

- 1.5 cups Raw Cashews soaked in water for at least 4 hours
- 13 oz coconut milk canned, full-fat works best
- 1⁄2 cup water
- 3 tbsp maple syrup
- 2 tbsp shredded coconut

Directions

- After soaking, drain and rinse the cashews.

- Place the cashews in a food processor or blender along with
the water, maple syrup, desiccated coconut, and coconut
milk. Process till smooth.

- After letting it sit in the refrigerator for about half an hour or
heating it on low for five minutes on the stove, serve.

7.BLOOD ORANGECELLO

Prep time:10 minutes
Cook time:20 minutes
Serving:8

Ingredients

- 2 cups vodka
- 5 blood oranges large • 0.5 cup sugar
- 0.5 cup water

Directions

- You should scrub the oranges to get rid of any wax on their skin before you start. After putting the oranges in a bowl of boiling water and letting them sit for a few minutes, clean them with a brush to get rid of any wax and then rinse them under colder water. After the oranges have dried, peel them thoroughly, making sure to remove most of the pith. Put the orange peels and vodka in a big jar, seal it, and let it in a cool, dark area for 48 hours.

- After the oranges are juiced, add the sugar and water to a medium-sized pot. After giving it a quick stir to dissolve, put it over high heat and boil it. Simmer the mixture for three minutes without stirring, or until it slightly thickens, then remove and allow it to cool.

- After straining the vodka to get rid of the peel, discard it. Pour the vodka and syrup mixture into bottles that have been sterilised.

- Serve on their own or together with club soda.

8.BLUEBERRY-WATERMELON BREAKFAST COCKTAIL

Prep time:3 minutes
Cook time:2 minutes
Serving:2

Ingredients

- 1 bottle Tsamma Watermelon Juice • 1⁄4 cup blueberries, fresh
- 1 lime sliced into 4 wedges
- 1⁄4 cup mint fresh leaves

Directions

- You can create two morning drinks with this recipe. Just cut it in half if you are only preparing one, and store the remaining Tsamma Watermelon Juice for later!

- Fill the bottom of two large drinking glasses with the mint leaves and fresh blueberries.

- Muddle the blueberries and mint gently to release their flavours. Use a wooden spoon handle in place of a muddler if you don't have one.

- After giving the Tsamma Watermelon Juice a good shake, divide it equally between the two glasses.

- Fill each glass with the juice from one lime wedge. Stir gently to mix.

- If preferred, garnish with extra mint sprigs and lime wedges.

9.AMARETTO SOUR COCKTAIL

Prep time:10 minutes
Serving:2

Ingredients

- 4 oz Amaretto
- 2 oz freshly squeezed lemon juice • 2 tbsp maple syrup
- ice
- sparkling water to taste
- lemon peel for garnish
- a dash of bitters optional

Directions

- In a cocktail shaker, combine the ice, lemon juice, maple syrup, and amaretto. Give it a good shake to blend.

- Divide between two lowball glasses after straining via a cocktail strainer. Add a squeeze of bitters, a wedge of lemon, and some lemon peel on top, along with sparkling water.

10.KALE SMOOTHIE

prep time:2 minutes
Serving:1

Ingredients

1 ripe banana peeled and frozen
1/2 cup frozen blueberries
2 teaspoons ginger peeled and finely grated 2 cups kale leaves loosely packed
1 cup unsweetened almond milk
1 tablespoon chia seeds optional
1/8 teaspoon ground cinnamon
2 teaspoons to 1 tablespoon raw honey

Directions

• In a blender, combine all the ingredients and process until fully smooth. If extra almond milk is needed to help your blender process the frozen fruit, add it.

CONCLUSION

As we wrap up our journey through the "Greenland Vegetable Cookbook," I want to express my sincere thanks for sharing this culinary adventure with me. It's been a pleasure exploring the world of healthy, delicious recipes with you, centred around my love for vegetarian diets, weight watching, and the sheer joy of eating well.

Final Thoughts:

What you hold in your hands is more than a cookbook; it's an invitation to embrace a lifestyle that cherishes your well-being without sacrificing the pleasures of taste. Each recipe is a small celebration, a reminder that the kitchen is a place of creativity, health, and connection with the food we eat.

Encouragement:

As you step into your kitchen, remember that cooking is an art, not a rigid science. Feel free to put your own spin on the recipes—tweak, adjust, and experiment. Your journey to a healthier lifestyle is personal, and every step you take in the kitchen is a positive stride toward a happier, healthier you.

Resources for Further Support:

To continue this journey beyond these pages, consider exploring nutrition guides, connecting with fitness communities, taking cooking classes, and diving into wellness blogs. These resources can offer additional support, inspiration, and knowledge to enhance your well-being.

As you move forward, know that your commitment to a healthier lifestyle is a continuous, evolving process. Whether you're a seasoned

cook or just starting out, may the "Greenland Vegetable Cookbook" be a companion in your pursuit of delicious, health-conscious living. Wishing you not only vibrant health but also countless moments of joy and satisfaction in your culinary adventures. Here's to your well-being and the delightful dishes that lie ahead!
Warm regards,
Yvette W. Messenger.

Review page

Dear Reader,

I hope this message finds you well! As the author of the "Greenland Vegetable Cookbook," I'm reaching out to kindly request your feedback. Your thoughts and

insights are invaluable in shaping the future editions and helping others discover the joys of healthy, delicious cooking.

If you've had the chance to try out the recipes or explore the content, I would greatly appreciate it if you could take a moment to share your thoughts. Your review will not only provide valuable feedback for improvement but also assist fellow readers in deciding if this cookbook aligns with their culinary preferences and goals.

Whether you loved a particular recipe, found a helpful cooking tip, or have suggestions for enhancements, your input is highly valued. Feel free to share your experiences and recommendations.

Thank you so much for being a part of this culinary journey. Your feedback is instrumental in creating a community of enthusiastic home cooks dedicated to savouring the richness of healthy, vegetable-centric cuisine.

Warm regards,

Yvette W. Messenger.